# What in the World
# are Organ Transplants?

# What in the World are Organ Transplants?

Written & Edited By:

Dr. Austin Mardon, Margaret Wa Yan Choi, Gurman Barara, Amy Li, Suad Alad, Christina McDonald, Julia Cara, Maryam Oloriegbe, Jasrita Singh, Tolu Atama, Sriraam Sivachandran, and Hafsa Alamagan

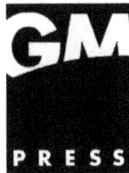

**GM**
PRESS

Cover and typeset by A. Boyd

Paperback ISBN 978-1-77369-247-0
Ebook ISBN 978-1-77369-248-7

GM
PRESS

Golden Meteorite Press
103 11919 82 St NW
Edmonton, AB T5B 2W3
www.goldenmeteoritepress.com

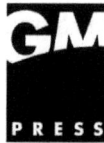

# Table of Contents

# Chapter 1:

# A Brief History of Organ Transplants

By: Margaret Wa Yan Choi

## Introduction to Organ Transplants

Organ transplantation is defined as the medical procedure that replaces a failing organ of the patient (recipient) with a healthy and functional one from an eligible donor (HealthLinkBC, n.d.; Shayan, 2001). This procedure is often conducted when one's organ functions are lost due to diseases or injuries and can be performed when the organ has stopped working completely or is no longer working well (HealthLinkBC, n.d.). Not all organs can be transplanted, and different countries have different regulations for the type of organ being transplanted (HealthLinkBC, n.d.). In general, the most commonly transplanted organs are the kidney, the liver, the heart, the pancreas, and the lungs (HealthLinkBC, n.d.).

Transplantation is not a simple procedure, and various factors need to be considered, a successful transplant can only occur under precise and well-defined conditions (Shayan, 2001). Organs and vessels must also be relocated and re-anastomosed or reunited accurately in order to ensure tissue and host viability (Shayan, 2001). In addition, to prevent infections and rejection of the donor tissues or organs, the immune system compatibility between the donor and recipient would need to be confirmed carefully (Shayan, 2001). A lot of sciences are involved in the process of transplantation, thus, it is considered a multidisciplinary science that encompasses fields of medicine, immunology, surgery, and anesthesiology, etc (Shayan, 2001).

## Myths and Legends about Organ Transplants

With organ transplantation being such a complex practice, one may think that it has been developed in more recent decades where there have been more advances in the field of medicine and technology. However, the concept of transferring body parts for healing or strengthening the body of the recipient is actually not new at all (Shayan, 2001). In fact, this fascinating idea had been suggested by humans from thousands of years ago, and descriptions of organ transplants as a miracle can be found in ancient or prehistoric myths and legends (Shayan, 2001). For instance, in Greek mythology, it is said that there were chimeric Gods and heroes with bodies formed from parts of various animals (Shayan, 2001). Many other examples can be found in the New Testament of the Bible, which states that Jesus was able to carry out autotransplant — transplant using parts that belong to the same individual — and restored a servant's ear after it got cut off by Simon Peter's sword (SAMU, 1960; Shayan, 2001). Also described in the Bible is the miracle brought by Saint Peter, who helped Saint Agatha reimplant her breasts that were pulled off during torture (Shayan, 2001). The Bible also states that a soldier's hand was cut off during a war, but was reimplanted by Saint Mark (Shayan, 2001).

The earliest records of an organ transplant can be dated back to the Bronze Age, a prehistoric period (Shayan, 2001). During this era, bone grafts were used on the sulls during trephination, which is the process that removes a circular disc of bone from the calvarium as an attempt to remove pressure within the skull (Shayan, 2001). This bone disc would then be placed back in the calvarium later, and this is considered an example of orthotopic autograft (transfer of a living part of the body) from the early times (SAMU, 1960; Shayan, 2001).

There are also records of ancient experiments with organ or tissue transplantation in archeological specimens found around the world, in places such as Egypt, China, and India (Shayan, 2001). The earliest known practice of skin grafting, which refers to skin transplantation, is recorded in the Ebers Papyrus, an ancient Egyptian medical papyrus that can be dated back to 1500 B.C. (Singh et al., 2017). Skin grafting was also highly developed in India, and there was a detailed description of this procedure written in Hindu text back in 700 B.C. (Shayan, 2001). According to the records, noses and lips could be reconstructed using grafts (epidermis and part of the dermis) containing skin and subcutaneous fat from the buttocks (Singh et al., 2017;

Ziegler et al., 2004). The knowledge and technique were brought to Europe and adopted by the ancient Romans and Greeks as well (Singh et al., 2017).

## Early Development of Organ Transplantation

In the later centuries, techniques in organ transplantation improved significantly (Shayan, 2001). In the 15th century, specifically during the 1590s, Gaspare Tagliacozzi, a well-known Italian surgeon, successfully used an upper arm flap to reconstruct the lost nose on his patient (Shayan, 2001). Historical records suggest that teeth grafting was performed on humans in the early 17th century (Shayan, 2001). Following is the 18th century, a time where a number of experiments with grafts from the skin, tendons, thyroid, nerves, cartilage, glands, ovaries, muscles, etc. were reported (Shayan, 2001). A Scottish surgeon named John Hunter conducted several transplantation experiments (Barker & Markmann, 2013; Setchell, 1990; Shayan, 2001). He transplanted human teeth and autotransplanted the cocks' spurs to the combs of the cocks (roosters), but the experiment did not succeed (Barker & Markmann, 2013). He later on experimented with transplantation of the testis (the male reproductive organ) of a cock into the belly of a hen (Setchell, 1990; Shayan, 2001). The testis adhered to the intestine, but it was believed that this did not affect the normal functioning of organs in the recipient (Setchell, 1990). This experiment involving testes was then repeated in 1785 (Setchell, 1990).

Experiments with transplanting different body parts or tissues continued in the 19th century (Shayan, 2001). In 1869, Jacques-Louis Reverdin, a Swiss surgeon in Geneva, discovered that small, thin grafts could be used in healing and would work better than larger grafts, he then developed the technique called "pinch grafts" to cover burns, ulcers, or open wounds (Barker & Markmann, 2013; Singh et al., 2017; Ziegler et al., 2004). This technique was later named "Reverdin pinch" (Singh et al., 2017). In this technique, implanted islands of epidermis acted as centers of epithelialization and growth on the wounds of the recipient (Singh et al., 2017). The first application of Reverdin pinch grafting was performed on a patient who had lost a portion of skin on his thumb. Two 1 mm$^2$ pieces of epidermis were placed on the granulation tissue on the patient (Singh et al., 2017). The development of Reverdin pinch grafting was a significant milestone in the history of organ and tissue transplantation. However, there were still several limitations. First of all, the grafts could cause contractures, which are fixed tightenings of the skin that restrict movements and reduce flexibility of the body part (Singh et al., 2017; Mayo Clinic, 2021). The grafts would also take quite some time to heal, and the new scar tissue was susceptible to stress and cosmetically unsatisfactory (Singh et al., 2017). Another famous incident of a successful allogeneic skin graft took place in 1898 (Shayan, 2001). During the Sudanese war, Sir Winston Churchill noticed that a fellow officer had a serious cut on his wrist, and so he donated a piece of skin from the inside of his forearm to help cover the wounds of his friend (Shayan, 2001; The Churchill Project, 2019). Throughout this century, surgeons and doctors were able to gain lots of valuable experiences and knowledge regarding autografts and homografts, prompting further discoveries in the future (Barker & Markmann, 2013).

## Development of Vascular Suturing for Organ Transplantation

The history of organ transplant is full of experiments, failures, and setbacks. Despite this, there were lots of valuable and pioneering work which laid a foundation for successful transplants in more recent decades (Hatzinger et al., 2016). For half a century, surgeons encountered lots of difficulties in conducting a successful homograft for kidney or other organ transplantations, and they found the homograft failure inevitable (Barker & Markmann, 2013). A turning point happened in the year 1902, when Alexis Carrel, a French surgeon, discovered a way to effectively perform vascular suturing—stitching and uniting the blood vessels of the new organ to those of its recipient (Barker & Markmann, 2013; Aida, 2014; Nobel Lecture, n.d.). Carrel himself had previously attempted to connect the blood vessels in a surgery, but wasn't satisfied with the results at all (Nobel Lecture, n.d.). He then went on to investigate principles for a new technique on human cadavers and performed vascular anastomoses, the joining of the blood vessels, on living dogs in collaboration with other professors and doctors at a laboratory (Nobel Lecture, n.d.). Through these different experiments, he was able to refine and modify the techniques (Nobel Lecture, n.d.). He noticed that the main cause of failures in past surgeries was the formation of blood clots (Aida, 2014). To overcome this barrier, instead of the large and thick needles that were traditionally used, he used atraumatic, small and round needles, and extremely fine sutures made of silk lubricated with Vaseline to stitch the vessels together (Aida, 2014). He also did not use a needle holder like the others, and chose to grasp the needle in his fingers (Aida, 2014). This required great dexterity and agility of the fingers, which he attributed to his lessons from Madame Leroidier, one of the finest embroiderers in France, as well as his repetitive practices of stitching on paper (Aida, 2014). At the end, Carrel was awarded the 1912 Nobel Prize for Physiology or Medicine in recognition of his work (Aida, 2014).

**First Successful Long-term Kidney Transplant**
The kidneys are two bean-shaped and fist-sized organs located below the rib cage, on each side of the spine (Mayo Clinic, 2021). They perform filtration and remove waste, minerals, and fluids from the blood by producing urine (Mayo Clinic, 2021). If their filtering functions are lost, fluids and waste would build up in the body, reach harmful levels and raise the blood pressure (Mayo Clinic, 2021). When the kidneys have lost about 85-90% of their ability to carry out their functions properly, one is said to have end-stage renal disease (Mayo Clinic, 2021; National Kidney Foundation, 2021). Some common causes of end-stage kidney disease are diabetes, chronic and uncontrolled high blood pressure, chronic glomerulonephritis (inflammation and scarring of glomeruli - tiny filters within the kidneys), and polycystic kidney disease etc (Mayo Clinic, 2021). At these stages of kidney failure, waste would need to be removed from the patient's bloodstream via dialysis, which utilizes a machine to

remove waste and extra fluids or salts, maintain a safe level of certain chemicals in the bloodstream, and control blood pressure (Mayo Clinic, 2021; National Kidney Foundation, 2021). However, dialysis does not cure the kidney disease nor recover the kidneys' functions (National Kidney Foundation, 2021). The most ideal solution to kidney failures is to get kidney transplant (National Kidney Foundation, 2021). Without a kidney transplant, one may have to undergo dialysis treatments for his or her rest of the life (Mayo Clinic, 2021; National Kidney Foundation, 2021).

In 1902, Emerich Ullman carried out the first successful transplantation of a dog kidney (Hatzinger et al., 2016). The kidney was connected to the arteries of the dog, and it did produce urine for a few days before the dog passed away (Hatzinger et al., 2016). Next, in 1909, more experiments with kidney transplants were carried out (Hatzinger et al., 2016). Efforts were made to transplant human kidneys from deceased patients to monkeys, other donors such as dogs, goats, lambs, and monkeys, were tried, but none succeeded (Hatzinger et al., 2016). In 1933, Yu Yu Voronoy, a Soviet surgeon, attempted the first human-to-human kidney transplant (Hatzinger et al., 2016). Unfortunately, due to improper handling of the organ, and a blood type mismatch, the surgery failed (Hatzinger et al., 2016). Later on in the 1940s, surgeons from other parts of the world continued experiments with dog kidney transplants (Barker & Markmann, 2013). For instance, Morton Simonsen in Denmark and William Dempster in London went on to actively carry out such experiments (Barker & Markmann, 2013). The outcomes were not desirable: no new insights were found, and it was advised that such surgical procedures should not be carried out on humans (Barker & Markmann, 2013). For a while, there seemed to be very little hope for successful long-term transplants in humans.

A huge milestone was reached later in the year 1954, when Dr. Joseph E. Murray collaborated with associates at Peter Bent Brigham Hospital (now Bridham and Women's Hospital) in Massachusetts to perform the first successful living donor transplant (United Network for Organ Sharing, 2018). The surgery was done with two twins, a healthy kidney was donated by Ronald Herrick to his twin brother, Richard, who was diagnosed with chronic kidney failure (United Network for Organ Sharing, 2018). After the transplant, Richard lived an active and normal life, and passed away due to causes unrelated to this transplant 8 years after (United Network for Organ Sharing, 2018). One of the main factors that led to its success was that the donor and the recipient were biological relatives, as this would reduce the risk of organ rejection and enhance the survival rate of the recipient following the transplant (United Network for Organ Sharing, 2018). According to other scientists or surgeons, in retrospect, this transplant was not as significant as it was said to be, since it had been known that rejection would not occur in skin grafts performed between identical twins (Barker & Markmann, 2013; United Network for Organ Sharing, 2018). However, this accomplishment was still indeed impressive as both the recipient and donor survived for a long time, its success also encouraged other surgeons to put in more efforts to explore organ transplants, resulting in the growth of this field, and of renal transplantations specifically (Barker & Markmann, 2013).

## Other "First" Successful Organ Transplants

Transplantation of other nonrenal organs such as the liver, heart, and pancreas was also starting to be explored and techniques kept getting refined (Barker & Markmann, 2013). Like kidney transplant, their success was also built upon lots of past experiments (Barker & Markmann, 2013; Júnior et al., 2015). In 1963, Thomas E. Starzl performed the first successful liver transplant, which was a surgery that no patient had survived previously (U.S. Department of Veterans Affairs, 2018). The patient passed away due to pneumonia several weeks after, but this was still considered a breakthrough and Starzl was regarded as the "father of transplantation" (U.S. Department of Veterans Affairs, 2018). In the same year, the first lung transplant was also performed (Health Resources & Services Administration, 2018). A patient that entered the emergency room died in shock due to a heart attack, the family allowed donation of the left lung for transplantation (Venuta & Raemdonck, 2017). James D. Hardy and his team then performed a transplantation with a patient that had a tumor in the left main bronchus (Venuta & Raemdonck, 2017). The recipient survived for 18 days following the surgery and died of renal failure and infection (Venuta & Raemdonck, 2017). Autopsy proved that the lung transplanted was well-ventilated and no evidence of rejection was observed, so overall it was considered a huge success at the time (Venuta & Raemdonck, 2017).

In 1967, the first human-to-human heart transplant was also

performed (Brink & Hassoulas, 2009). It was a challenging surgery performed by the South African surgeon, Christiaan Barnard, in Cape Town (Brink & Hassoulas, 2009; Cooper, 2018). One main challenge was that the recipient was far from ideal by today's standards (Brink & Hassoulas, 2009). The recipient was a 53-year-old smoker with severe coronary insufficiency, diabetes, and peripheral vascular diseases (Brink & Hassoulas, 2009). The donor was a 25-year-old who acquired a severe brain injury in a car accident and passed away due to brain death (Cooper, 2018). Soon after the donor was confirmed to have no chance of recovery and died, Barnard extracted the heart and proceeded with the transplant, while handling the heart carefully (Brink & Hassoulas, 2009). At first, the heart was not beating and there were concerns rising (Cooper, 2018). The surgical team wondered if the heart muscles had been severely damaged in the process (Cooper, 2018). Barnard applied electric shock to the heart and it started to contract weakly. Also with the help of a heart-lung machine, the heart beats became stronger and stronger (Cooper, 2018). In the end, the transplant was successful and the heart functioned satisfactorily (Brink & Hassoulas, 2009).


## Conclusion

Organ transplantation has had a long history. Today, with organ transplantation being a common procedure, it may be hard to imagine the difficulties the pioneers and surgeons had gone through in the past. As it is also viewed as an advanced surgical procedure, one may also find it surprising that the idea had already been born so many centuries ago. The journey of developing more advanced techniques for organ transplant continues, and it is hopeful that in the near future, the field will grow even larger along with the evolution of various techniques or technologies.

# Chapter 2:

# Origins of Organ Transplant Research

By: Gurman Barara

## Introduction

Organ transplantation is a significant advancement in medicine and an area of research that is constantly evolving. The concept of organ transplantation dates back centuries. For instance, Roman-Catholic accounts reported that the first ever leg transplant was performed by Saints Cosmas and Damian in the third century (Androutsos et al., 2008; Barker and Markmann, 2013). Although there are multiple reports of ancient occurrences of organ transplants and various myths and legends surrounding this phenomenon discussed in the previous chapter, there are several significant accomplishments over the past decades which have allowed for the modernization of organ transplantation. Several researchers and scientists have made groundbreaking advancements in the field of organ transplantation, a few of whom and their contributions will be discussed.

## Key Innovators and Contributors

Alexis Carrel, a French surgeon and Nobel Prize winner in 1912, is accredited with the development of vascular suturing and its implementation in organ transplants (Barker and Markmann, 2013). In the early 1900s, Carrel partnered with a physiologist named Charles Gunthrie in Chicago, where they successfully carried out whole organ transplants in animals (Cooley, 2002). Carrel's skill, use of fine needles and suture material, and aseptic technique led to his success with organ grafts and transplantation. During this time, Carrel had also claimed that the use of autografts—tissue retrieved from the same individual's body—are usually successful; however, the use of homografts— tissue retrieved from another individual of the same species— were not. This led to the exploration of why homografts did not work and the beginning of investigating whether there has to be a match between donors and recipients (Barker and Markmann, 2013). In today's date, determining whether there is a match between the donor and recipient is essential in organ transplantation. Another milestone achieved by Carrel is the development of the Carrel Patch, which is still a technique implemented in today's date (Vernon, 2019). Following World War I, Carrel worked alongside Charles Lindbergh to develop a device called a perfusion pump which was able to preserve organs for about three weeks. The device was initially designed to be used during open heart surgery but ended up being used to provide oxygenated blood to organs (Barker and Markmann,

2013). The device led to the development of modern day devices such as the pump oxygenator or the heart-lung machine (Redman, 2015). Carrel's research and discoveries in the field of organ grafting truly made him a pioneer in transplant surgery.

A contribution made by a German physician named Leo Loeb in the 1930s would go on to play a big role in transplantation research. Loeb was working at Washington University when he discovered that the rejection of skin homografts in rats was dependent on genetic differences between the donor and recipient (Barker and Markmann, 2013). Furthermore, Loeb also showed that lymphocytes (white blood cells) were involved in the body when skin grafts were performed. This suggests that the immune system plays a role in organ grafting (Barker and Markmann, 2013). This would later form the basis of immunosuppression therapy used following organ transplantation.

The first kidney transplant between humans was performed in 1933 by Yu Yu Voronoy. Unfortunately, the transplant failed, most likely because the kidney was retrieved six hours after the donor's death, and the kidney was not an appropriate match between the donor and recipient (Barker and Markmann, 2013).

William Dempster, a transplant surgeon and researcher in London, was involved in experimental trials of dog kidney transplantations in the late 1940s. Being familiar with some of Leo Loeb's work, Dempster implemented the use of radiation and the drug cortisone in organ transplant recipients (Barker and Markmann, 2013). The effects of cortisone increased the survival of skin grafts in rodents through immunosuppression effects

(Anderson et al., 1951). However, the use of cortisone and radiation in dogs did not suppress kidney rejection by the recipient. As such, Dempster advised against the use of this treatment in humans at the time (Barker and Markmann, 2013).

Since there was no effective therapy to prevent organ rejection, René Küss and David Hume started a trial program for human kidney grafts in Paris and Boston, respectively. During the time, patients with severe kidney failure had no methods of treatment such as dialysis (Barker and Markmann, 2013). Since patients with kidney failure were unable to receive effective treatment, the transplantation trial was allowed to be carried out. The Paris trial took place in 1951 and was led by Küss. The kidney grafts were performed retroperitoneally with a surgical connection of the renal artery to the internal iliac artery, the renal vein to the iliac vein and the ureter to the bladder (Cinqualbre and Kahan, 2002). All nine of the transplant patients died in a matter of a few days or weeks. It is worth mentioning that one of the patients received a donor kidney from their mother, which functioned at first but then ended up being rejected by the recipient in a few weeks (Barker and Markmann, 2013). The technique developed by Küss for kidney transplantations is the same method used in today's date (Cinqualbre and Kahan, 2002).

At the same time, David Hume led the transplantation trial in Boston. Hume carried out nine kidney transplants in which the recipients were treated with ACTH, cortisone and testosterone (Barker and Markmann, 2013). These drugs were used with the hope to suppress the recipients' immune response and prevent rejection of the donor organ by the body. Only four kidneys were functional for a brief period of time before failing. Surprisingly, one of the patients had a functional kidney for about six months until it was rejected (Barker and Markmann, 2013).

Based on the results of the kidney transplant trials led by Hume and Küss, it can be seen that all of the transplant patients ultimately died due to the kidney failure as the donor kidney was ultimately rejected. Ethics must also be taken into consideration when discussing this trial. Although the patients in the program were already experiencing renal failure and had no chance of recovery due to the lack of treatment at the time, it can be argued that it was unethical to conduct experimental trials on them. Moreover, the donor kidneys in the Paris program were retrieved from criminals who were executed (Barker and Markmann, 2013). This would raise an ethical debate in today's society as well: whether organs from death row inmates should be used in transplantation or not. There may have been a possibility that the kidney transplant would work, however, previous research and animal trials at the time clearly suggested that kidney transplantation was ineffective. Although the outcome of the trial itself was not a medical breakthrough, the subsequent events to follow led to significant advancements in organ grafting.

Peter Medawar was a British biologist who was working alongside Thomas Gibson, a plastic surgeon, to determine whether skin grafts would be a suitable treatment for burn victims (Barker and Markmann, 2013). It was found that homograft rejection occurred in patients due to an immunological response against genetically different grafts (Simpson, 2015). This explains why skin autografts (skin taken

from another part of the patient's own body) were not rejected—
there are no genetic differences. On the other hand, skin
homografts would be skin tissue taken from a donor and used to
treat a recipient. The genetic disparity between the donor and
recipient would have caused an immunological response to arise
in the graft recipient. Although Medawar concluded that organ
rejection is a result of an immunological response, he was unable
to detect any antibodies in skin homograft experiments in
animals (Barker and Markmann, 2013). Medawar later worked
alongside his colleagues, Hugh Donald and Rupert Billingham,
to carry out a skin graft between twin cows. Interestingly, most
cows would accept the skin graft from their twin with minimal
rejection. Medawar and his colleagues came to the realization
that cows likely accepted the skin graft from their twin because
of stem cell exchange in utero (Barker and Markmann, 2013).
Medawar then worked with Billingham and one of his students,
Leslie Brent, to minimize rejection in mice. Recipient mice were
injected in utero with donor spleen cells and about two months
after birth, the skin graft was performed. The recipient mice did
not reject the graft, which was transplanted from the
spleen donors (Brent, 1997). However, homografts from another
mouse, which was not the spleen donor, were rejected by the
recipient. This was a great advancement in transplant tolerance—the
concept of suppressing the immune system so it does not attack
organ transplants/grafts. Medawar was awarded a Nobel Prize for
this study in 1966 (Barker and Markmann, 2013). This study also led
to the discovery of graft-versus-host disease, in which donor stem
cells see the recipient's body as a foreign object and may elicit an
immune response (Brent, 1997). Organ transplantation tolerance and
graft-versus-host disease are still an area of research in today's date.

The first successful kidney transplant was performed by Joseph Murray. The recipient's identical twin was the kidney donor and thus, the recipient did not reject the kidney. Although it was already known that grafts between twins have been successful in the past and do not get rejected, this led to a spike in transplantation research (Barker and Markmann, 2013). The concept of injecting donor spleen cells in utero was not feasible in humans (Simpson, 2015). Thus, other methods to induce organ tolerance and minimize rejection had to be explored. Joan Main and Richmond Prehn were two researchers who showed that the use of radiation can weaken the immune system and then donor bone marrow cells could be introduced (Barker and Markmann, 2013). This became known as the Main-Prehn method and was used in 1958 by Murray and his colleagues. Only one out of the twelve patients survived—a patient who received a kidney from his fraternal twin brother (Barker and Markmann, 2013). This once again led to the thought that genetic similarity is required between the donor and recipient. However, in a few years this was shown to be untrue because Jean Hamburger and René Küss performed four transplant procedures in recipients who did not receive an organ from their twin. The grafts were performed with the use of total body irradiation, and donor bone marrow was not inoculated into the patients (Barker and Markmann, 2013).

**Immunosuppressive Drugs in Organ Transplantation** The use of radiation to suppress the immune system and prevent graft rejection was toxic and did not have a high success rate (Hurst, 2012). Thus, other approaches such as the use of chemical agents had to be investigated. Küss and Hamburger used drugs for immunosuppression in addition to radiation. One of the drugs administered to patients was 6-mercaptopurine (6-MP). The effects of such drugs in suppressing the immune response was studied by Robert Schwartz and William Dameshek (Barker and Markmann, 2013). Schwartz and Dameshek found that 6-MP extended the survival of skin homografts before it would be rejected by the recipient. Another surgeon, known as Roy Calne, investigated the effects of 6-MP in kidney transplants in dogs and found that the drug increased the survival of the kidney graft. This was the first successful use of chemical agents to suppress the immune system in transplantation medicine (Hurst, 2012). Calne pursued further research in organ transplantation and got a research fellowship with Joseph Murray. Calne also collaborated with George Hitchings and Gertrude Elion. Hitchings and Elion received a Nobel prize for the development of the immunosuppressants 6-MP and azathioprine—a derivative of 6-MP (Hurst, 2012). Calne found that azathioprine had a better therapeutic index and kidney rejection in dogs was delayed significantly through the use of this drug. As a result, azathioprine began to be used in human kidney transplants (Barker and Markmann, 2013).

In 1963, a conference was organized by the National Research Council. Some of the lead researchers in organ transplantation gathered in this conference to discuss kidney grafts. It was discussed that less than 10% of the kidney grafts patients survived for a period longer than three months (Barker and Markmann, 2013). The progress of immunosuppressive drugs was also discussed, which seemed only slightly more effective than radiation at that time. At the conference, a physician named Thomas Starzl discussed that when a chemical agent called prednisone is combined with azathioprine, graft rejection was minimized and even reversed (Hurst, 2012). Starzl was able to discover this when he was successful in reversing graft rejection in dogs through the combination of azathioprine and prednisone. The combination therapy of azathioprine and prednisone for immunosuppression became widely known and Starzl's method was adopted worldwide (Barker and Markmann, 2013). As a matter of fact, the success of this immunosuppressive therapy led to about 50 new transplantation programs being developed in the United States. Starzl also performed the first successful liver transplant through the use of refined surgical techniques and improved immunosuppression through the use of anti-lymphocyte globulin in addition to prednisone and azathioprine (Hurst, 2012). Due to his advancements in organ transplantation, Starzl was referred to as the "Father of Transplantation" (Eghtesad and Fung, 2017).

The use of azathioprine and prednisone was successful, and research in immunosuppressive drugs continued to grow. Calne began testing cyclosporine—a more potent immunosuppressive than azathioprine—in animal models and found an increase in kidney transplant survival (Hurst, 2015). However, in higher doses, the drug was found to be toxic, could lead to infections, and kidney failure. Similar to azathioprine, Starzl began to add prednisone to cyclosporine and discovered improved outcomes in kidney transplant recipients (Hurst, 2015). This became the standard immunosuppression therapy for transplant patients up until 1989, when Starzl showed the effects of tacrolimus.

Tacrolimus is a more potent drug than cyclosporine and minimized the rejection of the liver and other organ grafts that were resistant to standard immunotherapy treatment (Barker and Markmann, 2013).

## Brain Death

Up until the 1960s, the use of organs in transplants came from deceased patients. This limited organ grafting because once the heart stops beating, there are only a few minutes to remove viable organs before they get damaged due to a lack of blood circulation (Barker and Markmann, 2013). In the late 1960s, Harvard published that an irreversible coma or loss of function of the brain—also referred to as brain death—is accepted as death (Wijdicks, 2018). This publication was a controversial topic, especially for the retrieval of organs from brain dead individuals. However, the concept of brain death and the retrieval of viable organs from brain dead individuals became widely accepted; this also contributed to the rise in the number of organ donations and transplants (Barker and Markmann, 2013).

## Organ Preservation

In the early 1900s, Carrel and colleagues suggested that organs should be cooled for preservation. Organ preservation techniques were not used in the early stages of research and experimental trials; this likely contributes to the poor results that were obtained (Barker and Markmann, 2013). In the 1960s, the infusion of cold solution into the portal vein or renal artery was used for preservation of livers and kidneys, respectively. Preservation of kidneys ex vivo—outside of the body—through the use of a perfusion pump also seemed as an effective technique. This concept was similar to the perfusion pump developed by Charles Lindberg discussed earlier in the chapter. In 1987, the University of Wisconsin (UW) solution was introduced by Folkert Belzer (Barker and Markmann, 2013). Organs could be preserved by flushing the UW solution and cold storage. The solution contained agents that prevent cell swelling and stimulate normal metabolism (Southard and Belzer, 1995). Sometimes organs do not function properly when transplanted, and this may occur due to preservation related error and damage. It was found that continuous perfusion of kidneys with UW solution rather than cold storage could reduce preservation related damage (Southard and Belzer, 1995).

## Histocompatibility

Tissue matching for organ transplants was suggested by Carrel but was not feasible until Jean Dausset discovered the first human leukocyte antigen in 1958 (Barker and Markmann, 2013). The antibodies against the human leukocyte antigen were identified by Ross Payne and Jon van Rood (Barker and Markmann, 2013). Another physician, Paul Terasaki, developed a microcytotoxicity test which was able to identify donor specific antibodies and serum and reliably find optimal donor matches between family members (Barker and Markmann, 2013). Histocompatibility matching was an important finding and is still carried out in transplantation today to minimize rejection. The donor and recipient are matched according to their blood group and tissue typing; the recipient's blood serum reaction to donor cells is also considered (British Society for Immunology, 2017).

## United Network for Organ Sharing

The contributions of several transplantation researchers and physicians allowed for better surgical techniques, more efficient immunosuppression therapy to prevent rejection and overall, higher transplantation success rates. Until the 1970s, organ recovery and transplants were confined to individual hospitals (United Network for Organ Sharing, 2021). This means that if an organ wasn't available for the recipient at their hospital, there was no other way to locate suitable donor organs. The South Eastern Organ Procurement Foundations—an association composed of transplantation professionals in the United States— wanted to increase the efficiency of locating suitable organs for patients. The association launched a database in 1977 where the enrolled transplantation institutes would list their candidates to help locate a suitable organ. This database became known as the "United Network for Organ Sharing", or UNOS. A call centre to provide assistance with organ placement—now known as the UNOS Organ Centre—was also launched in 1982 in Richmond, Virginia (United Network for Organ Sharing, 2021). The National Transplant Act, introduced in 1984, stated that a national Organ Procurement and Transplantation Network be developed to coordinate organ transplant matches, and collect data about donors, candidates and recipients. In 1986, UNOS became the only organization to develop the requirements for this national network and has served as the Organ Procurement and Transplantation Network in the United States since then (United Network for Organ Sharing, 2021). The development of UNOS has allowed for efficient allocation of donor organs, a system to collect and analyse transplantation data and an increased amount of information provided to stakeholders of human organ transplants.

# Chapter 3:

# Impacts of Past Research
By: Amy Li

**Broadening What is Currently Understood**
**About Immunology**

Past organ transplant research played a significant role in the current understanding of immunology. In the history of organ transplantation, organ rejection between the donor and recipient was a serious matter. To ensure compatibility and blood-specificity between the donor and the recipient, scientists identified the red blood cell antigen groups carried by donors (Calne, 1994). Antigens are toxic substances that trigger an immune response in the body. Furthermore, scientists located these antigens in the major histocompatibility complex (MHC) (Calne, 1994). The MHC is a region of DNA that contains genes necessary for encoding proteins in the adaptive immune system. These antigens were class I MHC antigens, with most of them located in the liver (Calne, 1994). It is interesting to point out the liver since the liver belongs to secondary lymphoid tissue—a site that carries dendritic cells and other lymphatic cells that have not yet encountered antigens.

## The Field of Immunosuppression

Using the recipient's immune system to achieve a tolerance against the donor strengthened transplantation success. Immunosuppression has allowed scientists to understand the limits and boundaries of the immune system since severely weakening the immune system will kill the individual. It also introduced scientists to immunosuppressants—these are drugs that reduce immune activity (Calne, 1994). From the time that scientists postulated about injecting bone marrow from donors to support immune tolerance, researchers thought ahead in the field of immunosuppression (Calne, 1994). Factors such as the risk of infection and malignancy in the recipient were already considered with immunosuppressive drugs (Calne, 1994). An example is 6-mercaptopurine, a drug that targets leukemia: 6-mercaptopurine prevents rabbits from defending against outsider proteins (Calne, 1994). Transplantation mainly used immunosuppression to avoid organ rejection—this is achieved by introducing antibodies into the recipients (Calne, 1994). These antibodies eliminate lymphocytes belonging to the donor: such antibodies propelled the study of genetics (Calne, 1994). For example, scientists have found a low probability of MHC profiles being identical in siblings and to a greater extent between unrelated individuals (Calne, 1994). Nowadays, monoclonal antibodies are one of many immunotherapies used against different cancers; hence, without transplantation, the conception of injecting antibodies into patients may not have been used sooner.

Cyclosporine is an example of a drug used in immunosuppression; however, it caused nephrotoxicity in humans (Calne, 1994). To combat this problem, cyclosporine was distributed in lower doses or through a multiple-drug formulation, which consisted of a combination of steroids and other immunosuppressant drugs (Calne, 1994). The conception of combining other unique agents to create a more effective drug can be applied to the design of antibiotics or phage therapy; in antibiotics and phage therapy, multiple bacterium or phages can be combined to produce a stronger drug, using the strengths of certain compartments to makeup for weaknesses in others. Discovered in 1976, cyclosporine quickly became integrated into clinical medicine in 1984. The discovery of cyclosporine allowed scientists to explore other immunosuppressive agents that can reduce undesirable immune-resistant activity (Bezinover & Saner, 2019). Given its potential in preventing negative immune responses, the discovery of cyclosporine and similar immunosuppressive agents can set the stage for and help treat other autoimmune diseases, including arthritis.

Immunosuppressive drugs such as sirolimus prevent the mammalian target of rapamycin (mTOR), making them mTOR inhibitors. The discovery of mTOR inhibitors has also led to its potential to exhibit anti-tumour abilities. This ability is evident in patients who have grown tumours after transplant surgery (Watson & Dark, 2012). Therefore, immunosuppressive drugs and organ transplantation as a whole have a significant influence in targeting cancers and could be used in conjunction with other cancer therapies to maximize the treatment's benefit. An example of this is temsirolimus, an immunosuppressive drug that targets kidney cancer (Watson & Dark, 2012).

Designing immunosuppressive drugs and consequently avoiding organ rejection and toxicity has allowed surgeons to grow more comfortable with surgically experimenting with other organs, such as the heart, liver, and pancreas (Chang et al., 2004). It has also allowed scientists to be more creative with immuno-drug designs. For example, immunosuppressive drugs forgo steroids and calcineurin inhibitors: calcineurin inhibitors express immunosuppressive activity, leading to a reduction in T-cell activity. Instead, drugs will incorporate new agents such as alemtuzumab: alemtuzumab is also an immunosuppressive agent (Chang et al., 2004). Therefore, it avoids the deleterious effects of certain drugs (Chang et al., 2004). This type of thinking can also be applied to antibiotics; since bacteria gain antibiotic resistance, it makes sense to create new antibiotics that will target other bacterial cell wall components of resistant bacteria.

With such early exposure to immunology and exerted efforts to suppress immune activity, organ transplantation has leveraged current efforts in preventing the signalling cascades of T-cells in foreign organs (Chang et al., 2004). To ensure organ/graft approval into the recipient, T regulatory cells must regulate lymphocytes (T cells and B cells). This type of organ research has led to the study of cell treatment with T regulatory cells and how they ultimately lead to immune tolerance (Baan, 2018). For instance, scientists have found that T cells use different mechanisms for regulating immunological expression, such as through the demethylation of genes (Baan, 2018). Thus, organ transplantation has applications in cancer cell biology and cancer cell regulation.

Cells in innate immunity are also known to regulate the donor's immune cells; an example of this is myeloid-derived cells (Baan, 2018). Myeloid-derived cells inhibit T cells by activating T regulatory cells (Baan, 2018). This discovery is exciting and progressive in cell treatment, especially now that cell tagging of macrophages is available for use. With a better understanding of the activity of T cells, organ transplantation research has allowed scientists to use advanced technologies to build beyond their knowledge of T cells and humoral immunity. To conclude, organ transplantation research has enabled researchers to discover other unknown properties of innate or adaptive immune cells and use these findings towards enhancing existing immunotherapies against cancer or disease.

## Enhancing Surgical Technique

Organ transplantation research has also helped create surgical extraction methods. An example of this advancement is microvascular surgery—experimenting with organs near blood vessels (Dangoor et al., 2015). This detailed procedure requires the use of threads and delicate needles; however, with experience in grafting near arteries, organ transplantation made it less difficult for surgeons to handle small vessels (Dangoor et al., 2015).

Organ transplantation research also enhanced surgeons' knowledge of splitting liver organs. This surgical procedure is done according to the liver's lobes, an anatomical method for transplant and pediatric purposes (Dangoor et al., 2015). This knowledge can be applied to veterinary surgical procedures, enhancing surgeons' understanding of animal organ extraction. Moreover, the discovery of anastomoses, which connect adjacent channels, fibres, and networks in the body, has also made graft surgery easier (Calne, 1994).

## Emphasizing the Importance of Organ Preservation

Organ transplantation research emphasizes the importance of organ preservation and the specialized, controlled conditions that organs are kept in (Chang et al., 2004). The liquid in which organs are kept simulates intracellular conditions (Chang et al., 2004). In past research, scientists constructed a circulation system that shares many parallels with current perfusion systems for organ preservation (Jing et al., 2018). These developments led to extracorporeal membrane oxygenation and, later, perfusion systems for preserving organs (Jing et al., 2018).

Through dealing with transfusion liquids, organ transplant research helped scientists elucidate Xeno immunity; Xeno immunity is the body's inflammation or immune response to foreign species. The concept of xeno immunity came about when scientists mixed animal blood with human blood (cross-species blood), which they found was toxic to the organ (Jing et al., 2018). In addition, learning about organ preservation led scientists to understand the morphology of organs better, as well as the type of conditions organs should be kept in to ensure their quality (Jing et al., 2018). For example, organs controlled in cold blood may worsen organ damage, further weakening cellular metabolism or inducing spasms in the kidney (Jing et al., 2018).

Designing perfusion systems (perfusion is the flow of fluid through the circulation to an organ) such as *ex vivo* lung perfusion have inspired researchers to recognize the benefit of normothermic machine perfusion in other organ systems (Jing et al., 2018). This research made portable perfusion machines, opening paths for organ preservation while increasing its accessibility to the general public (Jing et al., 2018).

Advances in organ preservation have brought up the possibility of blood substitution in the future. These advances would mean using acellular oxygen carriers instead of human blood constituents that would share similarities to hemoglobin (Jing et al., 2018). This innovation would prolong organ preservation and inspire other fields of surgical medicine to incorporate these changes into their practice.

Organ preservation research has heavily impacted the field of tissue engineering. By using an "*ex vivo* machine perfusion as a platform, [tissue engineering] decellularized rat hearts by coronary perfusion with detergents in a Lagendorff apparatus, then reseeded these constructs by perfusion with cardiac or endothelial cells" (Jing et al., 2018, p. 852). Tissue engineering has even created bioartificial lungs in rats, implying a potential role of stem cells and perfusion as a promising field in organ engineering (Jing et al., 2018).

## Marking The Birth of Anesthesia

The birth of organ transplantation marked the start of anesthesia and critical care; unfortunately, this discovery was not as easily recognized (Bezinover & Saner, 2019). An important event was when a transplant surgeon, Dr. Antonio Aldrete, founded the post-anesthesia recovery score and created "the first prototype of the needle for spinal/epidural anesthesia but also performed anesthesia for the first liver transplant" (Bezinover & Saner, 2019, p. 2). Without anesthesia, this would hinder the success of organ transplant surgery, and surgical operations in general.

## Initiating Ethical Debates

Organ transplant research sparked the discussion of ethical debates associated with transplantation. The mortality rate associated with organ transplants and the sheer amount of donor deaths, often in young people, is daunting (Calne, 1994). To address this issue, transplanting gonads or the reproductive gland that makes gametes was a possibility at the time, but with it came many ethical considerations (Calne, 1994).

What is arguably the most considerable dying concern in this field is organ shortages. The recurrence and incidence of diseases also impact the state of organ shortages and research (Dangoor et al., 2015). Nonetheless, people will continue to rely on organ transplants; however organ transplant research findings have uplifted recent advances in stem cell research (Dangoor et al., 2015). In fact, since Starzl, an expert in organ transplantation, discovered xenografts, embryonic stem cells have been thought to have direct applications into organ transplants (Dangoor et al., 2015). Xenotransplantation and exploring the side of animals was considered yet thought to be an inaccurate field to delve into (Calne, 1994). However, xenotransplantation is now being incorporated into the field of organ transplant research.

## Impact on Psychological Research

The resurgence of psychological and neurological symptoms in transplant patients increases the demand for psychologists to be involved in transplant treatment (Rodrigue et al., 1994). The extent of psychological care depends on the transplant quality and whether there is evidence of an illness or indication of organ rejection (Rodrigue et al., 1994). In most transplant patients, these are just some of the areas of concern psychologists report depression and sexual dysfunction post-transplant (Rodrigue et al., 1994). While studying the clinical outcomes of organ transplantation in adult patients, it has been found that neurotoxicity or impairment occurs alongside the treatment of chemotherapy (Rodrigue et al., 1994). Given this type of consequence, researchers are interested in how neuropsychological effects impact the bone marrow transplants of patients (Rodrigue et al., 1994).

When studying the impact of organ transplants on the psyche, the concept of nonadherence in immunosuppressive drug treatment frequently appears (Rodrigue et al., 1994). Interestingly, in children, it has been shown that nonadherence in immunosuppressive drug treatment is correlated with higher emotional and informational support from fathers (Rodrigue et al., 1994). This finding can inform physicians on the secondary effects of organ transplant surgery on their young patients. The misuse of drugs can also be seen in antibiotics, where patients tend to not follow the course of their treatment.

When researchers consider all the possible factors affecting a transplant patients' recovery, organ transplant research has stressed the need to examine a patient's psychological status after any surgical procedure (Rodrigue et al., 1994). The research has also considered family situations or conditions that may affect the patients' overall psychological recovery process. The intersection between the two fields has also opened researchers' eyes to the methodological issues associated with organ transplantation, especially within the field of psychology (Rodrigue et al., 1994). Some of these methodological issues enhance ways to assess knowledge and understand the lack of reliability in measuring psychological status (i.e. interviews, symptom reports from patients themselves) (Rodrigue et al., 1994). In addition, prospective studies should be preferred over correlational studies to see the psychological effects over the course of the entire transplantation procedure (Rodrigue et al., 1994). Family member involvement is another factor within organ transplantation research that may impact the recovery process (Rodrigue et al., 1994). Since certain family members are required to be present during the transplantation process, this could harm the patient, especially if the relationship is toxic or unwanted (Rodrigue et al., 1994). Other factors such as the patient's social networks and the healthcare system they live under can heavily impact their recovery progress (Rodrigue et al., 1994).

Organ transplant research has taught medical professionals to look at the biological effects of treatment, and its holistic impact on patients' quality of life (Rodrigue et al., 1994). This conception enables researchers to work together with health economists to consider what variables are required to measure the quality of life (Rodrigue et al., 1994). Due to organ transplant research, integrating psychology into therapy and medicine can be possible (Rodrigue et al., 1994). This integration causes researchers to question the most beneficial forms of psychological therapy in organ transplantation: Is individual treatment most effective? Family therapy? Support groups? (Rodrigue et al., 1994).

In organ transplant research, the accuracy of psychological measuring tools in determining clinical outcomes has been debated, warranting further study (Rodrigue et al., 1994). For instance, there is a need for tools to differentiate between symptoms relating to the psyche, a comorbidity, a side-effect of a drug, or neurotoxicity due to another underlying disease (Rodrigue et al., 1994). There is also a need to choose patients undergoing similar medical conditions, making it easier to study and compare (Rodrigue et al., 1994). An example of this is organ transplant patients sharing parameters such as the severity of disease, disease type, and length of disease (Rodrigue et al., 1994). Lastly, confounding variables need to be explored further: age, gender, and how severely cognition has been affected in patients (Rodrigue et al., 1994). Given the wealth of knowledge taken from the intersection between organ transplants and psychology, more collaborative, multidisciplinary efforts are needed in the organ transplant research field to advance current knowledge, especially given the organ donor shortages and the impact organ shortages might have on future researchers' willingness to engage in the field (Rodrigue et al., 1994).

# Chapter 4:

# The Emphasis on Organ Research and its Growth Opportunities

By: Suad Alad and Christina MacDonald

**Importance Organ Research**

When it comes to obtaining, understanding and redistributing information regarding any topic, analyzing and researching are some of the best methods to consider. Researching a topic, especially for an extended period of time, allows for better comprehension of said topic, beyond what is commonly known or explained with surface-level understanding. In relation to organ donation and transplantation, in order to understand the processes of the procedures, the preoperative (pre-op) and postoperative (post-op) routines, and what is to be expected moving forward once the donation has been completed, one must understand the basics of organ research. With the help of organ donation, research on organ function can also lead to increased quality of life.

The process of organ research is done through organ donation, which can be conducted through methods of donation from patients that are either alive or dead. Known within the medical field, cadavers are one way organ donation research is performed on deceased bodies. Cadavers are always citizens who have consensually donated their bodies to medicine and are studied by medical students, physicians and other medical scientists to identify areas of disease or potential causes of death and allow for medical students to garner surgical practice (McCall, 2016). Research of the human body, and what it possesses, is crucial for the advancement of medicine for multiple reasons—to lead towards a better understanding of the human body, its healing process alongside treatments needed to facilitate this healing, as well as understanding the functions of each individual organ better. It is also an unfortunate benefit that, because these patients are dead, their ability to feel pain is nonexistent and allows for room for experimentation to be as invasive as necessary, within ethical boundaries.

According to the Physicians Committee for Responsible Medicine (n.d.), because there is no substitute for human tissue or the human body, donation is vital towards these methods of research and that whole-body donation (cadavers), is the best form of donation for this purpose. However, whole-body donation varies from country to country and is an extensive process to sign up for. Another form of organ donation conducted for research purposes is partial organ donation, however, it becomes a bit complicated based on what the patient is offering to donate. Similar to whole-body organ donation, partial organ donation is still a beneficial way to improve the understanding of the human body, but, because the donor is still alive, vital organs such as the heart, brain, both kidneys and entire lungs, livers and intestines, amongst other organs, are prohibited. Moreover, patients participating in partial organ donation are permitted to donate one kidney and part of their liver, pancreas or lung (Alberta, 2020).

## Methods of Research

### Deceased Organ Donor Intervention Research

The primary form of organ research is performed on whole-body donors and the use of organs donated by deceased donors has been found to "[…] identify new methods to improve the quality and increase the quantity of organs […]" that have the potential to be successfully donated and transplanted to recipients on the donor list (Liverman et al., 2017). With this method of research, the growing needs of the organs being donated and studied are addressed to improve organ donation quality through all stages of the transplantation process. The intent behind the research is to test methods of intervention that would otherwise make an organ no longer viable for donation during the transplantation process, assess this intervention and then curate potential alternative outcomes in order to keep all organs in the process of donation intact and thus increase the number of recipients awaiting a donation (Liverman et al., 2017).

The organs used during the process of this research are not only used for the research aspect but also have the potential to be donated and transplanted to recipients on a waiting list. Upon viability, once the research on each organ is conducted and it is concluded that the organs are successful for further donation, the organ is transplanted to a patient in need of it, providing the organs with a "dual purpose" (Liverman et al., 2017). Unfortunately, due to the ethicality of the procedures and the debate of bodily autonomy upon experimentation being called into question, this method of research is not as commonly used as most hospitals would like. Regardless, the intention behind the procedure is incredibly promising and provides great potential in the advancement of the process of organ donation. With this research, there is the potential for a donor to donate 8 of their organs (potentially 10 if their lung and liver are split in half), which maximizes the number of organs to be transplanted.

## Isolated Organ Research

Isolated organ research is the process of removing an individual organ and maintaining its physiological state for experimental and knowledge purposes (Knottenbelt, 2019). Unlike deceased organ donor intervention research, this method of study allows for researchers to maintain the organ's original physiological state for as long as needed because the experiment is occurring within a controlled environment. This way, external influence is limited and the optimization of gaining extensive knowledge of each organ is increased. For some organs, however, perfusion may be required for better results while the experiment is being conducted (ADInstruments, n.d.).

## Ethics and the Growth of Organ Research

In many places, there are strict ethics that must be followed when conducting scientific research. In Canada, for example, the Research Ethics Board was created to ensure that participants of all research are treated with respect and dignity at all times. Regardless of if the research is conducted with living participants, human remains, or specific tissue samples, one must follow ethical procedure (Government of Canada, 2021).

The first principle presented by the American Psychological Association under their General Principles section is the principle of beneficence and nonmaleficence. Although written for psychologists, ethical principles are transferable to any study. This principle speaks to how no harm shall be done and that it is imperative that the welfare of those involved is safeguarded (American Psychological Association, 2017). At first thought, it may seem difficult to imagine how organ research can be conducted without causing some harm; the organ transplant process itself could be considered harmful due to the fact that it is a surgical procedure that has the potential for error or rejection. Moreover, even though there is much more rigorous testing done on animals (which still follow ethical guidelines), the conclusions drawn from these animal models cannot be translated into definitive results for humans (Low et al., 2021). With new technologies rapidly advancing, scientists and engineers are refining the study of organs in a way that does not place human beings, or any animal, in harm's way.

A common issue found regarding the ethical implications of organ research is the invasive process of these procedures conducted throughout the studies. Methods of research like deceased organ donor intervention are seen as forms of research that do not respect the research participants because of the implication that the participants are seen as subjects of science before they are seen as human. Even though the donors used during the studies are in fact seen as human beings, because participants are having their physical bodies simultaneously studied and upon success, have their organs transplanted for donation, it begs the question of how human they really are in the eyes of the researchers (Liverman et al., 2017). These questions are asked even though the intentions behind the research are to maximize the use of the organs donated by these same participants and to decrease the potential for prolonged wait times through this maximization.

## An Incredible Advancement in Organ Research: Organs-on-Chips

Studying mini-organs for scientific advancement—being able to compile a sort of database of all the different cell types, their functions, their reactions to chemicals, diseases, drugs and various other factors—may sound more like a plot for a dystopian movie rather than a tangible scientific advancement, but this technology is already being utilized today.

Organs-on-chips, also called microphysiological systems or 'tissue chips' is a fairly new technology that holds great potential for medical and pharmacological discovery and advancement in relation to organ research (Low et al., 2021). These chips are helping to eliminate the need for animal testing by providing an alternative way to understanding the function of many different organs through microscopic cross-sections of human tissues (Wyss Institute, n.d.).

These chips are made of a clear, flexible polymer material, and are comparable in size to a memory stick (USB) for a computer. There are channels within the disk that are lined with the specific cells; these cells are very specific to what organ is being studied (Wyss Institute, n.d.). Different variables can be altered within the chip to simulate different bodily functions and environments depending on what type of cell is being studied. For example, if there is a lung cell, the chip can simulate breathing using vacuum channels to see how the cells react. Scientists can introduce bacteria into the created 'airstream' and see how the 'bloodstream', specifically how the white blood cells (which attack invading cells) react in response (Wyss Institute, n.d.). Enhancing the view of the three-dimensional structure of the cells as well as different forces that impact the movement and biomechanics of the various cells types is crucial (Low et al, 2021). The complexities of the physiological processes that can be studied are great and have the potential to continue to advance.

Organs-on-chips can have significant implications in understanding disease, drug delivery, and may even help reduce drug development costs (Wyss Institute, n.d.; Woods, 2017). As the chips can emulate various environments, being able to test different drugs on various cell tissues and conditions can greatly impact transplantation medicine. Even though the focus is often placed upon the procedure of transplantation, organ recipients must take anti-rejection medication. A challenge with the development of anti-rejection medication, which are immunosuppressant drugs—drugs that suppress the body's natural immune defence system so that the transplanted organ is not flagged and attacked—is that they may have toxic effects on the immune system (Provincial Health Services Authority, n.d.; Shanti et al., 2018). With many drugs failing clinical trials due to toxicity, it is extremely beneficial to be able to test the drugs on chips, especially those with human cells, to be able to reduce overall and better predict the outcomes that will be seen in clinical trials (Shanti et al., 2018).

## Body-on-chip

Further growth is possible moving from organ-on-chip to body-on-chip. This would entail using different organ chips in tandem, to simulate more complex biological function (Boettner, 2020). Being able to better conceptualize the links between the different biological tissues and mechanisms is an extremely promising advancement that can directly impact the understanding of organ donation and transplantation.

## Who Does Organ Donation Research Help? How?

### The Patients on the Waitlists and Their Socioeconomic Implications

The people affected the most, both positively and negatively, by organ donation and its research are the patients who are in need of these donations. But who are these patients and just how affected are they by organ donation and the donation waitlists?

According to the National Kidney Foundation (2016), as of 2014, the race of the patients that made up both majorities for patients who received as well as donated their kidneys in the United States is Caucasian/White. Similar statistics were found in the U.S. Government Information on Organ Donation and Transplantation website (2021), which states that approximately less than 50% of Americans in need of organ transplants actually receive, but that out of every racial identity, White patients still make up the majority of both patients who donate their organs, and patients who need organs donated.

Neither website suggests or comes to the conclusion that People of Colour (PoC) are inherently more healthy than White people or that they are less likely to require organ donations. The U.S. Government Information on Organ Donation and Transplantation website actually makes it a point to address that race is not a factor in the donation needs or process, but that having a diverse list of donors makes for access to donation better for racialized groups, as donation can depend on location and community (Health Resources and Services Administration, 2021).

## So Why Do PoC Make Up Such a Small Percentage of These Statistics?

A major reason, and one that needs to be considered going forward, is that many PoC living in the West do not have universal access to healthcare and cannot afford to go to the hospital for medical treatment. In Canada, communities that are racialized make up the country's statistical majority for who is amongst low-income communities (Government of Canada, 2019). This implies that access to medical centres and hospitals is scarce and thus decreases the potential for routine check-ups and can lead to the reduction of catching organ failure or infections early on. This could also imply that PoC living in the West are dying before they can even consider getting on a donor list and that because they do not have access to basic methods of health and medicine, the options of considering becoming donors prior to dying decreases as well and their organs are not donated once they are proclaimed dead.

## How Diversifying Organ Donation Research Can Help?

With the advancement of organ donation research, considering the statistical differences in racialized versus White citizen's access to information regarding organ donation can lessen the discrepancies between these groups. A glaring issue in why PoC make up such a small percentage of donation statistics is that they are unaware of the options or opportunities in the first place. Without access to basic information about organ donation, consideration for their needs in the research process regarding said donations becomes just as scarce as their access to these procedures, and more lives are lost than saved as a result. Thus, their inclusion in the research must become mandatory.

Race and ethnicity do not play a deciding factor in the probability of successful matching between a donor and a recipient. However, because blood compatibility and tissue make-up is more common between people of a shared racial or ethnic group, donors of every race are beneficial in the racial accessibility for organ donation (LifeSource, 2021). The consideration and inclusion of races beyond those who are White can and will save the lives of millions moving forward. In order to do this, diversifying the research conducted for organ donation *is* crucial and needs to be an affirming factor as the advancement of organ donation research ascends towards a promising future.

## There is Still Room For Growth

Science is dynamic. There will always be room for growth in the various scientific fields; especially when it comes to the medical sciences and organ research, there is still much to learn about what needs to be done to improve the quality of human life and how to do it. Even with the ethical standards that must be followed, in this highly technological world, there is great opportunity for advancement without risking any human lives. Moreover, as this world is diverse and impacted by a multitude of interconnected systems, it is important that there is some level of interdisciplinary collaboration and intersectional analysis, even in specialized fields of medical sciences, to further reach these findings. As technology and collaborative research continue to advance, so will the scope of organ research, who it affects and the real-world implications that follow.

# Chapter 5:

# Medical Procedure of Organ Transplantation
By: Julia Cara

## The Basics

To better understand this chapter, it is important to have a clear understanding of some of the medical terminology used in organ transplant literature. This chapter will focus on organ transplantation, beginning by defining the broader categories of tissue transplantation. Keep in mind skin—a type of tissue—is the largest human organ.

Tissue transplants can be grouped into four main types: allograft, autograft, xenograft, and domino transplant. When most people hear the word "transplant" they think of transplants which occur between a donor and a recipient. In this case they are really talking about allografts, defined as the "transfer of tissue between genetically nonidentical members of the same species" (Corfield, n.d.). Allografts make up a large percentage of the world's transplants, but include many risks, such as organ rejection (Nasr, 2016). Autografts, the transplantation of tissue from one part of the body to another in the same individual, is uniquely immune to rejection because the genetic material is identical to the body and therefore is not identified as "foreign" by the immune system. Autografts are often used in reconstructive surgery where skin, bone, nerves, blood vessels, or tissue is removed from one site on the body and returned somewhere else. The third type of transplant, xenografts, involve an interspecies tissue or organ transplant, for example porcine (pig) heart valve transplants (Manji, 2012). Finally, domino transplants are a series of transplants, performed consecutively, in which a patient is both a donor and recipient. For example, when cystic fibrosis (CF) patients receive a lung transplant, it is often easier to transplant both the lungs and heart of a deceased patient into the CF patient at the same time (Cochrane, 1991). The CF patient becomes the recipient of a new and healthy set of heart and lungs but is also able to donate their healthy heart to another patient.

Further classifications can be made depending on the donor: live organ donors, donation after brain death, or donation after circulatory death (He, 2018).

## Deceased Donation

Though millions of people around the world are registered as willing organ donors, very few people—only three in every thousand deaths in the United States—die in a way that allows for organ donation (HRSA, 2018). In order to become a deceased donor, one must die under very specific circumstances;one that maintains the health and viability of the potential donor organs. Often, deceased donors enter the hospital after a stroke, brain aneurysm, or an accident which causes severe head trauma (HRSA, 2018). Despite the best efforts of a medical team, trauma to the head or brain damage due to strokes and aneurysms can lead to brain death.

Brain death is most clearly defined as "the irreversible loss of all functions of the brain, including the brainstem" with the three critical or defining characteristics being a coma, the absence of any brainstem reflexes, and apnoea—the absence of voluntary breathing (Goila, 2009). In other words, brain death means that a person can no longer breathe independently, nor do they display any brain activity. Being an irreversible condition with no hopes of recovery, brain death has long been considered a true "death" by both the medical community, religious leaders and the general public for many decades (Goila, 2009). Important in this context, a diagnosis of brain death is the first crucial step in the deceased organ donation process (HRSA, 2018).

Once a prospective donor is officially pronounced deceased, the hospital notifies the local Organ Procurement Organization (OPO) to confirm their donation candidacy (HRSA, 2018). Depending on the province or state, organ donation can be authorized immediately if the patient had been a registered organ donor, or by next of kin if the family agrees or believes the person would have wanted to donate. The donor patient is then matched with recipient patients.

## Living Donation

Though most organ donations come from deceased donors, living donations make up about a third of all yearly transplants. Living donors are usually related to the recipient, either a family member or friend, although some people choose to donate to someone they don't know—aptly named an altruistic living donor (HRSA, 2018).

For obvious reasons, living donors are limited in what organs they can donate. The most common are kidney donations, as it is quite possible to have a good quality of life with only one kidney. Liver donation is another option, as the liver is a regenerative organ, meaning that the donated lobe of liver will grow back. It's also possible to donate a lung (or part of a lung), part of the intestines, or part of the pancreas (HRSA, 2018). Blood, platelet, and serum donations are also considered living tissue donations.

## Organ Viability

The entire organ transplantation process runs on a very tight schedule. From the moment the donor is pronounced deceased, a countdown clock begins. While recipients are being matched, the donor's body remains on life support where it is being artificially oxygenated (HRSA, 2018). However, once removed from the body, organs have a limited healthy lifetime. For this reason, though a patient may spend months or even years on a transplant waiting list, their surgery must take place within hours of a matching organ becoming available. Due to time restrictions, most organs go to patients in close geographical range of the donor patient, though some are able to travel further.

Depending on the organ, viability can last between 4 hours and 36 hours (Lanese, n.d.). Hearts are most sensitive to a lack of blood flow, and the likelihood of complications with a transplanted heart increase dramatically after the 4 hour mark is surpassed (Lanese, n.d.). More resilient, the lungs can remain viable for 6 to 8 hours and the liver for up to 12. Kidneys, the most commonly transplanted organ, can remain viable for up to 36 hours.

Viability is fundamental in organ transplants. The function of the organ—or "primary graft" as it is often referred to in literature — both in the short and long-terms depends on ischemia–reperfusion injury (Bellini, 2019). Ischemia-reperfusion injury is the cellular dysfunction and death that occurs when blood flow is restored to ischemic tissues—ischemia being a condition in which blood supply does not meet a tissue's demand (Cowled, 2011). Most organ damage occurs in the time between retrieval and implantation. Organ preservation attempts to lower the level of ischemia-reperfusion injury to the cells of an organ by inducing hypothermic conditions to slow the cells' rate of metabolism and reducing oxygen usage.

The three primary preservation techniques are static cold storage, hypothermic machine perfusion, and normothermic machine perfusion (Bellini, 2019). Static cold storage is the current standard practice for kidney transplants and involves storing the organ on ice. Hypothermic and normothermic machine perfusion both involve flushing the organ with fluid before and during storage, the greatest difference between them being the temperature of the fluid—either 4°C or ~30°C (Kay, 2011). Static cold storage is favoured for its simplicity and low cost, however, several studies have shown that hypothermic machine perfusion reduces complications and is superior to static cold storage, particularly with deceased donors (Bellini, 2019; Tingle, 2019).

Throughout the matching and procurement processes, the donor's body is maintained on life support—artificial respiration and circulation which keeps the organs oxygenated—and the vital signs of each organ is monitored (HRSA, 2018). Once the organs have been matched to recipients, the donor's medical team—the team which was involved with the donor's previous care—is replaced by a surgical transplant team (HRSA, 2018).

## Recovering Organs

Disclaimer: the surgical techniques used for multi-organ procurement have evolved and been refined over the decades. The following descriptions are generalized steps in an incredibly complicated process and not comprehensive. The information contained in the following paragraphs – if not otherwise referenced – is informed by the 2018 article written by He et al. entitled *Procurement of Abdominal Organs in Multi-Organ Donation in Deceased Donor.*

The donor patient's body is prepared in a similar fashion as all other surgeries. The area is shaved, sterilized, and draped so that the surgical field is ready for the first incision. Depending on the organ(s) being donated, the proper incision is made and the transplant team examines the organs to rule out any malignant diseases (He, 2018).

In multi-organ procurement there are two phases: the warm dissection and the cold procurement (He, 2018). The warm dissection involves dissecting the tendons and vessels of each organ under normal circulation, while the heart is still beating. The cold procurement involves all those removed post pericardiectomy (removal of the heart).

The distal aorta is the first thing to be dissected and tied off. The liver is then freed by dissecting (or dividing) the left triangular ligament, hepato-gastric ligament, and the hepato-duodenal ligament. Donor arteries supplying these organs are preserved as much as possible so that they can be grafted to recipients' arteries. Following the dissection of the liver, the pancreas is left partially exposed and is the next organ to be dissected. The gastrocolic and gastrosplenic ligaments, which connect the stomach to the transverse colon and spleen respectively, are divided.

The pancreas is then assessed for transplant suitability. If suitable, the spleen will be dissected alongside the pancreas. Including the spleen in the pancreas transplantation is thought to help mitigate the chances of graft rejection, one of the two primary causes of failure in pancreas transplants (Booster et al., 1993). However, results are inconclusive as to the efficacy of the theory in practice (Booster et al., 1993).

Very rarely is the small intestine a donated organ. However, when it is, it is dissected after the pancreas. The ends of it are marked for future orientation and the arteries which supply it are saved. Finally, the aorta is dissected again, this time at a location just beneath the diaphragm. At this stage the warm dissection is finished, and the cardiothoracic team is substituted in to begin the heart and lung dissection and removal. Once the heart and lungs are removed, a cold perfusion line is set up and inserted into the aorta which was previously dissected. An ice slush is also applied topically to the abdominal region to cool the body through external means. This process takes approximately 20 minutes.

Cold procurement usually begins with the removal of the liver, however if the small intestine (which was previously dissected) is being removed, it will be taken out first. The pancreas can be removed after the liver, or with it 'en bloc'. Removing the two (liver and pancreas) en bloc helps to minimize ischemic injury to either organ. Finally, the kidneys are removed last and can be removed separately – the right one first, followed by the left – or en bloc and separated later.

After all the major organs are removed, any additional tissues that the family has authorized to be donated – such as bones, corneas of the eyes, or skin – are removed (HRSA, 2018). All incisions are surgically closed, and the procurement process is considered finished.

## Transporting and Transplanting Organs

The organs are placed in three different sterile bags, which is then placed on ice (He, 2018). The transplantation process begins once the surgeons and organs arrive at the hospital where the recipient had been prepped. The new organs are then grafted into the recipient. The length of the surgery will depend upon the organ being transplanted.

## Face Transplants

Perhaps one of the most fascinating transplants, which truly demonstrates the life changing effects of these surgeries, are face transplants. The first human face transplant was that of Isabelle Dinoire in France in 2005 (Lanchin, 2012). Dinoire received a new nose, mouth, and chin and news of her successful operation spread worldwide. Face transplant technology and procedures have evolved in the decades since her ground-breaking surgery, and in 2020 Joe DiMeo received the world's first face and double hand transplant (Simko-Bednarski, 2021).

Face transplants are one of the most complex of all transplant surgeries, can last more than 16 hours, and require the coordination of more than 100 medical professionals (Johns Hopkins, n.d.). Finding a match for a patient is extremely difficult, and can take months. A great number of criteria are considered including skin colour, gender, race, and the size of the face or features (Johns Hopkins, n.d.).

The toll of the surgery and recovery, both physically and psychologically, requires candidates to undergo extensive screening. Not only does the candidate have to be healthy enough to have the surgery, but they must prove that they are willing and able to follow the carefully crafted recovery regimen (Johns Hopkins, n.d.). That regimen always includes taking antirejection medication and going to physical therapy to begin learning how to use their new facial features. Personality and emotional resilience are also assessed. The road to recovery for face transplant recipients does not end with their surgery. If anything, that is where it starts. Recovery is a long process that can take anywhere from four to six months as patients relearn how to speak, blink, swallow, smile, and eat again (Johns Hopkins, n.d.). For this reason, patients must show an ability to overcome adversity and the inevitable stumbles as they make progress towards their goals. Having a strong support system is crucial.

The transplant itself mirrors that of other transplants, except that the surgeries are performed simultaneously (Johns Hopkins, n.d.). Incisions are usually made in places that are less noticeable, like near the hairline and below the jaw, but ultimately depend on how much of the face is being transplanted. Once both the recipient and donor are prepared, the face is placed onto the recipient. The bones are connected first using metal plates and screws. Arteries, nerves and veins are then sutured together with a surgical microscope and tests are performed to ensure that blood flows to all of the new tissues (Johns Hopkins, n.d.). With time, new networks of blood vessels will form, further connecting the donor and recipient skin. Once that critical step is successful, all the other muscles are connected, and the skin is sutured up.

## Transplant Rejection

Despite the efforts of all medical professionals – from the matching and procurement team, to the transplant and recovery team – sometimes a patient's body will reject a transplant.

There are three types of rejection: hyperacute rejection, acute rejection, and chronic rejection (Medline Plus, n.d.).

Hyperacute rejection occurs when the antigens of the donor and recipient are not properly matched. An example of this is when a patient with type B blood is given type A blood which is incompatible. This rejection becomes obvious just moments after the organ is transplanted. The transplanted tissue must be removed immediately or there is risk of death to the recipient.

Acute rejection occurs in the days and weeks following transplantation (Justiz Vaillant, 2021). The immune system recognizes the transplanted organ as foreign and attempts to attack it. The difference between acute rejection and hyperacute rejection is that hyperacute rejection occurs due to the presence of preformed antibodies, whereas acute rejection occurs due to antibodies which take time to develop – hence the delay in rejection (Justiz Vaillant, 2021). Immunosuppressive drugs are used to prevent rejection, and transplant patients (save those who receive autografts) must take anti-rejection immunosuppressive drugs for the rest of their lives.

Finally, chronic rejection is a manifestation of the body's immune response which occurs over many years and slowly damages the transplanted organ (Medline Plus, n.d.). It is characterized by "vasculopathy, fibrosis, and atrophy of graft with progressive loss of function that culminates in graft loss" (Gorantla, 2010). Vasculopathy is a blood vessel pathology, while fibrosis is the formation of scar tissue and atrophy is the reduction in tissue size. Chronic rejection leads to organ failure and the organ(s) will have to be removed and replaced.

## Conclusion

Organ transplantation is a complex process which requires immense coordination and serendipitous circumstances. The matching process is essential to preventing acute rejection, and the care of the procurement processes determines the quality of the organs. Though transplant medicine comes with high risks, the reward is the gift of life.

# Chapter 6:

# The Journey of Transplantation Sciences

By: Maryam Oloriegbe

## Introduction

Organ transplantation seems nothing much of a far-fetched idea: it requires taking out a failed organ to replace it with a functional one; however, in reality, organ transplantation is one of the most scientifically complex concepts in the world of medicine today. Immunology, among other sciences, has contributed to ensuring transplantation is as feasible as possible as many lives are saved from this medical innovation. Additionally, it is essential to acknowledge how and why organ transplantation can work in relation to different disciplines of science. This allows for a better understanding of why factors related to organ transplantation such as organ rejection, high blood pressure, and infection can occur and why physicians and researchers can avoid them as much as possible.

**Improving Organ Transplants throughout time**
Organ transplantation has come a long way since the first skin transplant in 1869 (Timeline of Historical Events and Significant Milestones, 2018). One of the most notable transplant surgeries to date is grafting, a surgical procedure in which one tissue is moved from one body part or one organism to another without moving the blood supply in hopes that the tissue grows its own blood supply. The practice of free skin grafting began in the 19th century in association with anastomosis, the surgical connection of two structures, this case being two blood vessels. Surgical anastomosis was developed in 1911 and is still being developed further and used today (Calne, 1994). As for skin grafting, surgeons Jacques-Louis Reverdin, George David Pollock, Louis XEL Ollier, George Lawson, Carl Thiersch, Fedor Krause, and Reissberg Wolffe used the theories and attempts of previous pioneers to successfully use free skin grafts in humans (Ang, 2005). Reverdin experimented and improved epidermal grafts in 1869, with Pollock later using his case study to do an epidermal graft on an eight-year-old suffering from burns on her thighs. In the 1870s, Wolffe and Krause developed full-thickness grafts involving the epidermis and the dermis, later publishing a case study in 1875 and naming the successful discovery of the Wolffe or Wolffe-Krause skin graft. With Lawson and Ollier also making discoveries of full-thickness skin grafts and other developments, the surgical field has seen a boom in innovation and improvement of free skin grafting. "From the establishment of the first Skin Bank in 1944, to an ever more detailed

understanding of the role of the immune system, and to the use of cultured and tissue engineered skin grafts, the developments of the 20th century have changed the field" (Ang, 2005).

Another standard example of organ transplantation that is common, especially in patients with kidney failure, is kidney transplants, the removal of a failed kidney in replacement with a functional one from either a living or deceased donor. These surgical procedures can be life-saving and very complicated given the recipient and the donor's pre-surgical procedures. To determine if the functional kidney will be a match, the recipient's blood and tissue type must match with the donor's; a cross-match must also be done to ensure the donor's cells can mix successfully with the recipient's blood serum. Failure to pass all three tests results in the ability for a kidney transplant to take place, and the recipient must wait for another kidney that matches. The first kidney transplant was done in 1936 by U Voronoy, but unfortunately, it failed, as did many early transplants in the 18th century. In 1960, in the UK, Sir Michael Woodruff and Mr. James Ross performed the first successful kidney transplant on twin boys (History of Kidney Transplantation, 2018). Both lived for about six years before dying from an unrelated disease, suggesting that replacing a damaged kidney can give the recipient a better quality of life and longevity. In 1962, the first kidney transplantation between unrelated patients (everything done before had been with siblings or parents and their children) was done using immunosuppression to reduce the chances of rejection of the kidney (Barker & Markmann, 2013). Previous surgeries had not used immunosuppressant drugs, making this specific surgery unique due to the advancements in the understanding of the kidney and how the immune system reacts in the presence of a foreign organ.

Organ transplantation has been occurring since as early as 2500 years ago (Ang, 2005). Physicians and researchers have come a long way to recognizing the importance of this surgical procedure and the life-saving qualities associated with it. Today, organ transplantation is performed on almost all organs and parts of the human body. Much more research is being done to improve the technique associated with the procedure and minimize the risk factors that follow with transplanting an organ, such as rejection, infection, and many more complications.

## Synthetic Biology and Focused Areas of Improvement

Rejection is a major complication associated with organ transplantation. Researchers have been attempting to control it at both the molecular, genetic and cellular level, but "the scale and complexity of the modifications required have made engineering of cells and organs for transplantation extremely difficult" (Stevens, 2016). However, synthetic biology has helped make large-scale mammalian genome modification possible and successful.

Each organ has a different response to rejection, although the immune mechanism may be similar. Researchers have focused on broad areas to improve when addressing modifications and transplantations (Stevens, 2016).

## Controlling Rejection Mechanisms

Both adaptive and innate immune responses have pathways where each step is interdependent; controlling one step may have broader effects on the entire outcome of a specific response or even a multitude of responses. For example, inflammation from phagocytic immune cells will activate the complement system and coagulation. Tissue damage from this will further release more stimulators that can further activate innate and adaptive immunity. Controlling key points early on in the pathway will ensure a reduction or elimination of damage of the donor cells and tissues, halting the synergistic activation of other pathways that can lead to rejection of the organ.

## Increasing Tolerance

An organ or cell's ability to provoke an immune response "can be altered depending on the form of antigen presentation, the microenvironment, and regulatory molecules to induce or suppress responses to a given antigen" (Stevens, 2016). Different modifications use the existing mechanisms in the immune system and alter them to increase the tolerance to donor tissues. This is especially desirable when considering the side effects of immunosuppression drugs and other complications, including risks of infection and tumour formation (Stevens, 2016).

## Cell Biology and Regenerative Medicine

Cell biology has played an essential role in organ transplantation, specifically within regenerative medicine, the process of replacing or regenerating human cells, organs, or tissues to restore normal function. There are various ways in which regenerative medicine can occur to aid in the feasibility of organ transplantation.

## Cell Therapy

Cell therapy is defined as the injection of cellular material into a patient. The injection itself can either be human cells from a donor to a recipient, such as with neural stem cell therapy and hematopoietic stem cell transplantation or injecting animal materials to cure disease (Jain & Bansal, 2015). The first practice has strong potential and has shown significant results with many conditions such as osteogenesis imperfecta, myeloid malignancies, and Hurler's Syndrome (Jain & Bansal, 2015). The second practice has not been proven effective and can result in severe consequences (American Cancer Society, 2008 as cited in Jain & Bansal, 2015).

## Generation of Organs Using Adult Stem Cells Generating

organs from a single stem cell purified from the tissue has shown promising results. Researchers were able to generate mammary glands using isolated single stem cells from the mammary glands of an adult mouse (Shackleton et al., 2006 and Stingl et al., 2006 as cited in Jain & Bansal, 2015). Scientists also reported that a single stem cell from the epithelial lining of a mouse prostate generated a functional prostate (Leong et al., 2008 as cited in Jain & Bansal, 2015).

## Organ Printing

Organ printing is a new emerging technology that is described as a process by which layers of "additive robotic biofabrication of

3D functional living macrotissues and organ constructs using tissue spheroids as building blocks" (Mironov et al., 2009 as cited in Jain & Bansal, 2015). It typically involves three steps; development of blueprints for organs and digitization of the image of the organ or tissue is obtained, layered processing of the actual organ by placing cells into a 3D environment; and passing blood through the blood vessels of the organ and accelerated organ maturation (Jain & Bansal, 2015). Bioprinting has had some success with many organs, as one scientist performed a mechanical fabrication of living trileaflet heart valves using valve cell populations and 3D printing (Duan et al., 2013 as cited in Jain & Bansal, 2015). Currently, scientists are working on bioprinting kidneys, bladders, and hearts. However, a significant limitation to this technique is that the organs tend to only live for a couple of days at best (Thomas, 2015 as cited in Jain & Bansal, 2015).

## Immunology of Organ Transplantation

The immune system is a highly biological complex system whose responsibility and function is to differentiate particles that are host and non-host, which can be further characterized as foreign. The immune system's effector mechanisms, immunological memory, and ability to destroy microorganisms and foreign particles make it the body's most robust defence system. Unfortunately, the immune system can work a little too well and enable the rejection and attack of organ transplants from allogeneic sources.

As mentioned previously, a donor and recipient must go through three primary tests to determine whether the donor's organ will be a match for the recipient. If one or more of these tests fail, the organ can not be transplanted. However, even after passing all three tests, the recipient's body can still reject the organ. For this to occur, the transplanted tissue must be recognized as foreign by the immune system. Subsequently, effector mechanisms are activated and attempt to destroy the tissue. The process by which the immune system identifies a foreign tissue is allorecognition, and its subsequent responses are known as the alloresponse. Tissue antigens are molecules on the tissue that are capable of stimulating an immune response. Many different types provoke an alloresponse, but the three antigens that exist on tissues are ABO blood group antigens, human leukocyte antigen (HLA) antigens, and non-HLA antigens (minor histocompatibility (MHC) antigens).

ABO blood group antigens are glycoproteins found on red blood cells and other tissues involved in blood vasculature, such as the endothelium. The blood types that exist include A, B, AB, and O, and each type has its own unique properties. Individuals with Group A have Antigen A on the surface of their red blood cells and develop anti-B antibodies; individuals with group B have antigen B on their red blood cells and develop anti-A antibodies. Thus, if a patient with a blood type of B received 'A' blood, the anti-A antibodies would respond by destroying those red blood cells. The opposite also occurs for blood group A. Interestingly, AB patients have both A and B antigens on the surface of their red blood cells and develop no antibodies. This gives them the ability to receive blood from any blood group, making it the universal recipient. Blood group O has neither A nor B antigen and possesses anti-A and anti-B antibodies and can not receive blood from any other blood groups except another individual with O type blood. A, B, and AB blood groups can receive blood from O blood groups, making it the universal donor. Because the anti-ABO antibodies develop from the start of childhood and are pre-existing before the time of transplantation, a mismatch in blood types between the transplanted organ and the recipient can result in a "rapid activation of the complement system and [organ] loss in almost all organ types"(Chandak & Callaghan, 2014). Although essential, compatibility of ABO blood groups, however, is not a significant barrier to transplantation,

In contrast to ABO blood group antigens, HLA antigens play a significant role in organ transplantation as they are the main target for an alloresponse. They are cell-surface proteins whose responsibility is to "present small portions of proteins (peptides) for recognition by receptors of cells of the immune system" (Chandak & Callaghan, 2014). HLA antigens are encoded by the genes found in the major histocompatibility complex (MHC), a region on the short arm of chromosome 6 in humans (Chandak & Callaghan, 2014). There are two main classes of HLA antigens: Class I and Class II, each of which have different roles. MHC Class I molecules present peptides (degraded proteins) from intracellular proteins of pathogens or self-proteins. MHC Class II molecules receive the degraded proteins and present them to either B or T cells to destroy the particle. Within both classes, many subtypes differ by the degree of polymorphism and have many different variations within the subtypes. The diversity across HLA antigens is thought to prevent susceptibility to a specific pathogen and are therefore highly immunogenic. Unfortunately, this can have drastic consequences for organ transplants in terms of the alloresponse provoked by the antigens on the foreign HLA antigens on the tissue. Furthermore, "as HLA class I and II molecules are widely expressed on a variety of cell types, they can act as tissue antigens in transplanted organs, even though their biological function is entirely different" (Chandak & Callaghan, 2014).

## Non-HLA antigens

Though their significance in organ transplantation is thought to be minimal, hence called minor histocompatibility antigens, they can still act as transplant tissue antigens. As non-HLA antigens on allogeneic tissues show variation through some degrees of polymorphism between individuals, their peptides are considered to be immunogenic and will be presented on HLA class I and II molecules, later recognized by the recipient's immune system.

## Immunosuppression and Tolerance

Immunosuppressive drugs are used to subdue or prevent the immune system from aggressively reacting to specific antigens on tissues. Depending on the class, their mechanism of action varies but includes preventing lymphocyte activation, the proliferation of immune cells, and downstream effector mechanisms (Chandak & Callaghan, 2014). They act non-specifically, meaning that they suppress the immune system due to the organ transplant and infectious agents and neoplastic cells, thus increasing the risk of infections and other side effects associated with the drugs (Chandak & Callaghan, 2014).

Tolerance is defined as the lack of antigen-specific immune response without the need for immunosuppressants which are drugs. It is often described as the 'holy grail' of transplantation because of the prevention of an alloresponse and elimination of immunosuppressive drugs and their potential side effects (Chandak & Callaghan, 2014).

## Rejection

Rejection is the immune system's response to a foreign object, the organ transplant, and the process it undergoes to damage it. It can occur anytime after transplantation occurs but typically occurs after the first year. There are usually different types of rejections, and each type has different times of onset or times when they typically happen.

Hyperacute rejection typically occurs within minutes to a few hours. The mechanism by which it occurs is as follows: pre-formed antibodies (anti-HLA or anti-ABO) are usually present in high volumes, and all attack the organ attempting to destroy it (Chandak & Callaghan, 2014). This action activates the complement system or complement cascade, in which factors in the immune system enhance the activity of antibodies and phagocytic immune cells to destroy the foreign object or particle, initiate inflammation, and attack the object's cell membrane. This, unfortunately, leads to cell destruction, organ thrombosis (formation of blood clots within the vessels supplying blood to the organ), and necrosis (body tissue death).

Acute rejection occurs within weeks to a few months, and it typically is cell-mediated and/or antibody-mediated. In a cell-mediated attack, macrophages, T cells, and neutrophils within the organ attack it, causing its damage. In an antibody-mediated attack, anti-donor antibodies (antibodies that fight the donor organ) produce B cells which initiate the complement system and the further degradation of the organ (Chandak & Callaghan, 2014). Differentiating between the two is difficult as they both have the same effects on the organ; however, histological features and detection of anti-donor antibodies in the recipient serum is one method of examining the difference.

Lastly, chronic rejection typically occurs within months to a few years and can be cell or antibody-mediated and occurs via chronic or long-term, alloimmune responses. "Chronic low-level immunological responses combined with hypertension, immunosuppressive toxicity, hypercholesterolemia, underlying donor disease, and age-related changes are known to result in slowly progressive graft dysfunction" (Chandak & Callaghan, 2014).

## Conclusion

The sciences that have contributed to the advent of organ transplantation have improved and paved the way for further development and innovation in the field. Understanding how the immune system works with immunology has allowed scientists and researchers to understand rejection and other complications at a molecular and cellular level. Synthetic and cell biology in association with regenerative medicine has helped modify and alter specific immunological and cellular pathways that aid in reducing the probability of transplanting a failed organ.

# Chapter 7:

# Challenges in Organ Transplantation

By: Jasrita Singh

## Introduction

Organ transplantation is a life-saving procedure for patients affected by terminal organ failure. In most cases, receiving a transplant from a donor is the only option to life for these patients. This vital procedure is accompanied by several challenges that limit its therapeutic potential.

## Organ Shortage

Owing to the increasing incidence of end-stage organ failure and growing success of solid organ transplantation, the demand for donor organs has been rapidly rising. However, the supply of the vital organs remains insufficiently low. As a result, the list of the number of people waiting to receive an organ transplant and those dying waiting for one is becoming longer by the day. As of February 2021, more than 107,000 individuals are on the national transplant waiting list in the United States of America alone. A whopping 90% of adults in the United States support organ donation, however only 60% are actually signed up. This disparity is concerning and closing this growing gap is imperative. In the United States alone, 17 people die each day waiting for an organ transplant, with the need for a donor kidney being the highest, followed by the liver, heart and the lung. Every 9 minutes a person is added to the transplant waiting list, and the rate at which a person is removed from the list is insignificantly low (Organ Donation Statistics, 2021). This widening gap is the greatest challenge facing the field of organ transplantation today, and is one that is claiming thousands of lives each year.

## Allograft Rejection

The advent of organ transplantation was limited by the inevitable risk of allograft rejection during its initial years of discovery. Allograft rejection is a consequence of the recipient's immune system response to the foreign antigens expressed by donor organs. The three major types of allograft rejection are categorized as hyperacute, acute, and chronic rejection (Kloc & Ghobrial, 2014).

**Hyperacute rejection** begins within minutes or a few hours after the transplantation and is arguably a result of the most severe and violent immunological reaction . It is caused by the presence of preexisting antibodies, in the recipient's blood, that are directed against the donor (Moreau et al., 2013). The immune response leads to severe inflammation and induces irreversible damage of the allograft. Fortunately, existing screening methods to detect anti-donor antibodies eliminate a majority of the hyperacute rejection cases, and their presence is considered an absolute contraindication to transplantation (Kloc & Ghobrial, 2014).

**Acute rejection** occurs within the first few weeks to several months post-transplantation and affects every transplanted organ to a varying degree. The activation of the immune system leads to uncontrollable inflammatory response and the death of the allograft tissue (Moreau et al., 2013). Currently, post-injury allograft biopsy is the gold-standard in diagnosing acute rejection. Given that the biopsy yields a diagnosis after the allograft has been injured warrants the discovery of non-invasive biomarkers to identify early signs of acute rejection (Nasr et al., 2016). Nevertheless, as a preventive treatment, intense immunosuppressive therapy is a standard-of-care in organ transplantation and has resulted in a marked decrease in acute rejection cases. Immunosuppression serves as the basis of modern day organ transplantation, which has resulted in long-term survival and meaningful functional recovery of many patients (Black et al., 2018). With current prescription of immunosuppressants, the one-year graft survival rate now exceeds 90%. This is in stark contrast to the early days of organ transplantation, where survival was limited to a few weeks (Sandwijk et al., 2013). However, the use of these drugs does not come without its own share of side effects. Prolonged use of immunosuppressants can lead to severe outcomes, such as an increased risk of post-malignancies (cancer) or the contraction of infectious diseases. For instance, the most common malignancies among transplant recipients are non-melanomatous skin cancers, affecting nearly 1 in 4 of liver transplant recipients (Unlu, 2015). The risk of infectious diseases is further discussed in detail. The use of immunosuppressive drugs in transplantation is one of the contributing factors to the shortened life expectancy of transplant patients (Duncan, 2005). *Sometimes the decision boils down to a choice between two evils, and the lesser of the two evils is chosen!*

**Chronic rejection** develops within months to years post-transplantation and largely caused by accelerated arteriosclerosis - hardening of the arteries or graft vasculopathy - progressive narrowing of graft vessels. This results in ischemia, which is a deficiency of blood, and hence oxygen, reaching a tissue as a result of the constriction or obstruction of local blood vessels (Moreau et al., 2013). The onset of ischemia, accompanied by incessant, prolonged immune system responses results in cell death and graft failure. There is no effective treatment for chronic graft rejection and efforts remain concentrated towards preventing episodes of acute rejection as a method to retard the progression to chronic cases (Kloc & Ghobrial, 2014). In many situations, the current standard-of-care for chronic rejection patients is retransplantation, which is less than ideal especially considering the ongoing organ shortage crisis (Biswas Roy et al., 2018). Current research in finding personalized approaches to treating chronic rejection is underway.


## Increased susceptibility to infectious diseases

With prolonged immunosuppressive therapies playing a predominant role in the direct prevention of acute graft rejection and an indirect role for chronic graft rejection, it is essential to consider the challenges posed as a result of its use. Immunosuppressive agents used in solid organ transplantation not only reduce the risk of allograft rejection, but also increase the susceptibility of organ recipients to common infections or those caused by opportunistic and obligate pathogens (Welte et al., 2019). Animal studies have shown that the host responses and the pathology of infectious diseases are strongly influenced by the type of immunosuppressive regime that is prescribed (Balloy et al., 2005).

## Bacterial Infection

Immunocompromised patients, including solid organ transplant recipients, are highly susceptible to common and opportunistic bacterial infections. This is largely due to the weakened ability of the immune system to defend against pathogenic bacteria as a result of reduced number of white blood cells (also known as leukocytes). Neutrophils are a type of leukocytes that comprise the first line of host immune response against invading bacterial pathogens (Witter et al., 2016). In patients undergoing immunosuppressive therapy post-transplantation, the development of neutropenia is a common occurrence in many types of organ transplants, especially kidney transplants. Between 20-50% of kidney transplant recipients experience neutropenia - an abnormally low number of neutrophils in the blood (Mavrakanas et al., 2017). Transplant recipients can contract bacterial infections in one of four ways - during the transplantation operation, during post-transplantation hospitalization (nosocomial infections), during active immunosuppressive treatment, and in the months occuring after the operation, when the immunosuppressed individual resumes normal life (e.g. community acquired infections) (Patel & Paya, 1997). Nosocomial infections in solid organ transplant recipients are approximately 20 times more frequent than in transplantation patients. Furthermore, solid organ transplant recipients are three times more likely to be admitted to hospitals from emergency departments (Timsit et al., 2019). Bacterial infections are the leading cause of infectious diseases in transplant recipients, accounting for infections in 33-68% of liver transplant recipients, 21-30% of heart transplant, 35% of pancreas transplants, 47% of kidney transplant, and 54 % of lung transplant recipients (Patel & Paya, 1997). Increased likelihood of contracting a bacterial infection, coupled with a weakened immune defense system, often leads to transplant recipients experiencing severe bacterial infection outcomes, including sepsis, allograft damage, and death. Sepsis is a life-threatening clinical pathology characterized by the body's extreme response to an infection in the blood caused by a pathogenic bacteria (Centers for Disease Control and Prevention, 2021). For the past several years, sepsis has consistently remained the first or second cause of mortality among all types of allograft recipients, affecting 20-60% of all transplant recipients and in-hospital mortality ranging from 10-40% (Kalil et al., 2018). Potent antibiotic treatments are used throughout the transplantation process as prophylaxis, during the surgery to prevent surgical site infections and post surgery to treat post-transplantation (De Simone et al., 2020). The growing prevalence of antibiotic resistance is threatening the ability to conduct these life-saving procedures.

**Fungal Infection**

Invasive fungal infections post-transplantation continue to be a significant cause of morbidity and mortality in solid organ transplant recipients. Despite groundbreaking improvements in therapeutic and diagnostic tools, consequences of post-transplant fungal infections can be severe and result in long hospitalizations, allograft damage and high death rates (Shoham & Marr, 2012). Host pathophysiology and environmental factors are vital determinants in the likelihood and severity of fungal infections in transplantation. These epidemiological factors include previously quiescent fungal infections, post-transplant environmental exposure to pathogenic fungi, use of antifungal prophylaxis (a pre-emptive prescription of antifungal treatment without confirmation of infection) and the state of immunosuppression (Shoham & Marr, 2012). Recipients or small bowel transplants are at the highest risk of developing fungal infections at 11.6%, followed by lung (8.6%), liver (4.7%), heart (4.0%), pancreas (3.4%) and kidney (1.3%) transplants (Pappas et al., 2010).

Candidiasis, a fungal infection caused by the *Candida* species, is the most common invasive fungal infection accounting for 50-60% of all fungal infections occurring after solid organ transplantations (Silveira & Husain, 2007). A recent study found the overall annual estimated incidence of candidemia in solid organ transplant recipients to be more than 13 times more likely than other hospitalized patients (3 vs 0.21 per 1000 admissions) (van Hal et al., 2009). The second most common infection is aspergillosis and is response for 20-25% of fungal infections. In lung transplants recipients, aspergillosis is the most commonly occurring fungal infection (Neofytos et al., 2010). Exposure to this fungal infection is almost exclusively due to the inhalation of *Aspergillus conidia* from an environmental source, and as a result, infection nearly involves pathology of the respiratory tract and/or sinuses (Shoham & Marr, 2012). Invasive fungal infections are highly prevalent in immunocompromised and chronically ill transplant patients and those requiring hemodialysis, high levels of immunosuppressants retransplantation being at the highest risk (Gavalda et al., 2005). In addition, treatment of patients with resistance to antifungal medications is more complicated.

Donor-derived fungal infections are becoming an increasingly recognized mode of transmission, where the transplanted organs may act as reservoirs for pathogenic fungi (Ison et al., 2009). Though active fungal disease in the donor is a contraindication to organ transplantation, latent infection unknown to the donor or transplantation team may result in the transmission of the fungal infection from the donor to the recipient. In addition, unexplained symptoms in the donor may only result in a diagnosis after the transplant recipient exhibits symptoms of fungal infection (Shoham & Marr, 2012).

## Viral Infection

Solid organ transplant recipients are at a high risk of developing clinical illnesses, often with increased severity, as a result of common and opportunistic viruses. These viral infections may be acquired in three different ways: donor-derived infections, community-acquired infections or from the reactivation of endogenous latent virus (Cukuranovic et al., 2012).

Herpes viruses, specifically cytomegalovirus and Epstein Barr virus, are most common opportunistic viral infection-causing pathogens in solid organ transplant recipients that are commonly transmitted with the allograft (Singh & Limaye, 2015). Symptomatic cytomegalovirus infection is evident in 20 to 60% of all transplant recipients and is a major cause of increased morbidity and mortality in this population (Brennan, 2001). Interestingly, the incidence of cytomegalovirus infection is considerably low in renal transplantation recipients at 8-32%, partly due to the lower burden of latent virus in the renal allograft. The highest risk for the development of viral infections is between one to three months post-transplantation, as immunosuppression is the greatest during this time (Azevedo et al., 2015). A study conducted in 2004 showed that both symptomatic and asymptomatic cytomegalovirus infections were independent risk factors for overall mortality in patients 100 days post-transplantation and reduced allograft survival (Sagedal et al., 2004). The Epstein-Barr Virus infects nearly every human before adulthood, and the infection is largely asymptomatic in childhood. Once infection occurs, the immune system develops a defence against the virus, which is maintained for life (Cukuranovic et al., 2012). However, iatrogenic immunosuppression post-transplantation to reduce the change of allograft rejection results in the failure of the immune system to defend against the Epstein-Barr Virus infection. This leads to a heightened risk of developing a wide range of life-threatening malignancies, including posttransplant lymphoproliferative disorder (Styczynski et al., 2008).

Community-acquired respiratory virus infections, such as those occurring from the adenovirus and influenza viruses, are a common cause of clinical disease and hospitalization in solid organ transplant recipients. These infections can lead to upper respiratory tract disease, but transplant recipients are at a significantly higher risk of complications occurring in the lower respiratory tract (Manuel et al., 2014). Adenovirus, for instance, can additionally result in complications including gastroenteritis, cystitis, and necrotizing hepatitis. In immunocompromised transplant patients, adenovirus infections tend to be more prolonged, severe, and may cause fatality (Cukuranovic et al., 2012). Moreover, influenza infections can occur at any time after the transplantation procedure and appear to be most severe within the three month posttransplantation period. The risk of contracting influenza infections is the highest in lung transplant recipients, followed by kidney and liver recipients (Manuel et al., 2014). Treatment of respiratory viral infections involves supportive care, and for influenza infections, oseltamivir or zanamivir are prescribed as treatment for both influenza A and B (Cukuranovic et al., 2012).

## Protozoan/Parasitic Infection

Parasitic infections lead to serious complications in solid organ transplant recipients, although their prevalence is lower than bacterial, viral and fungal infections. Owing to the increasing number of immunosuppressed transplant recipients, increased immigration and travel to and from developing countries, and increased attention directed to diagnosis and publication of these cases, the reported prevalence of parasitic infections has been on the rise in the past decade (Schwartz et al., 2013). Other contributing factors include transplant tourism - patients from developed countries undergoing transplantation procedures in endemic areas and returning with acquired parasitic infections, transplant individuals leisurely travelling to endemic areas, donors with latent or asymptomatic parasitic infections being referred to transplant centers in Western countries etc (Babik & Chin-Hong, 2015; Fabiani et al., 2018). The severity of the clinical presentation of parasitic infections largely depends on the features of the parasite, innate and acquired host immune, and the immune interaction between the parasite and the host (Schwartz et al., 2013).

A large number of serious post-transplant parasitic infections are protozoan infections caused by protozoa which establish lifelong latency in the donor or the recipient. These species have the ability to transform into lethal opportunistic infections in immunosuppressed, post-transplant patients (Halawa et al., 2019). One such infection is toxoplasmosis, a life-threatening zoonotic illness caused by infection from the protozoa *Toxoplasma gondii* (Furtado et al., 2011). A study found that post-transplant toxoplasmosis transmission occurred through infected allograft in 31.5%, de novo infection in 9.9% and reactivation of latent infection in 8% of infected recipients. The modality of infection in 50.6% patients remained unknown. Primary toxoplasmosis acquired through the allograft was found to be about 4 times more severe than the reactivation cases, with allograft toxoplasmosis leading to 31.4% death and reactivation mortality rate being 7.7% (Fabiani et al., 2018). Heart transplant infections are riskier than other solid organ transplant related toxoplasmosis, with the most common method for transmission in transplantation being through latent infection in the donor heart (Khurana & Batra, 2016). Toxoplasmosis occurs globally but is more prevalent in endemic regions, including France and the tropic areas of Latin America and sub-Saharan Africa, where the prevalence may approach 90% (Robert-Gangneux & Darde, 2012). Prophylaxis measures and extensive pre transplant screening is performed in these regions and has yielded largely successful outcomes. A multicenter, matched case-control study conducted with 15 800 solid organ transplant recipients in 11 spanish hospitals revealed 22 cases of toxoplasmosis. The median time of diagnosis following transplantation was 92 days, and the crude mortality rate was 13.6% or 3 of the 22 patients (Fernandez-Sabe et al., 2011). Although uncommon, toxoplasmosis (and other such protozoan diseases) in solid organ transplant recipients cause substantial morbidity and mortality (Fabiani et al., 2018).

## Conclusion

Organ transplantation is a life-saving process that provides meaningful functional recovery for many throughout the world. However, the therapeutic potential of this procedure is limited by significant challenges including organ shortage, risk of rejection and the spread of infectious diseases post-transplantation. The continued success of organ transplantation necessitates the development of novel strategies to mitigate such challenges.

# Chapter 8:

# Controversy of Organ Donorship

By: Tolu Atama

**Introduction**

Organ transplantation has been around for some time now. It is the removal of an organ from one part of the human body to another part. Usually, it is from a deceased person but it can sometimes be from a living person. It is often used to save lives especially when the only chance for survival involves transplantation. Kidney, heart and liver transplantation have been successful especially kidney transplantation (WHO, 2021b).

The purpose of transplantation can be medical or aesthetic related. Despite the success rate for life saving transplant procedures, some people still have a negative perception of organ transplantation. Nevertheless, these procedures must follow legal and ethical processes including obtaining consent (WHO,

2021b). Even though these ethical principles are followed, controversies still exist because unethical methods are sometimes used to obtain the organs—for example, when vulnerable donors are involved (WHO-A, 2021).

## Epidemiology

Globally, the need for organ transplants outweighs the availability of organs or organ donors. The data obtained from more than one hundred countries across the globe show that more than a hundred thousand organ transplants are performed annually. Of which about 70,000 was kidney transplant – about a half of this number was from living donors. About 20,000 from liver transplant – of this number about 20% was from living donors. More than 5000 was allotted to heart transplants; about 3500 and 2500 was allotted to lung transplant and pancreas transplant respectively. Over 20,000 donors were reported to have been from the deceased (WHO, 2021a). In the United States closer to 40,000 transplants were performed in 2020 and more than 100,000 people were on the waitlist as of the first quarter of 2021 (Organ Donor Statistics, 2021).

In Canada, the rate of obtaining an organ from a living donor remained the same compared to the rate ten years ago. However, the rate for obtaining an organ from a deceased donor increased by about 60% within a decade. Over 3000 transplants were performed with an increase of above 40% in the past 10-years. Comparable to the United States, there are quite a number of people on the waitlist for organ transplantation, with kidney transplants having the highest number both on the waitlist as well as the transplanted list (CIHI, 2020). This indicates that kidney transplants are more in demand and are the most performed procedure of all organ transplants in both the United States and Canada. There has been an increase in the rate of end-stage kidney disease in Canada, therefore, the demand for organ donors for the transplant procedure is increasingly high.

## Table

Organs transplanted, waiting lists and deaths on waiting list, by organ,
Canada including Quebec, as of December 31, 2019*

| Organ type | Number of organs transplanted | Number of patients on waiting list | | Number of patients who died on waiting list |
|---|---|---|---|---|
| | | Total | Active | |
| Kidney | 1,789 | 3,299 | 1,902 | 72 |
| Liver | 610 | 526 | 412 | 107 |
| Heart | 212 | 142 | 88 1 | 8 |
| Lung | 404 | 237 | 186 | 41 |
| Pancreas | 68 | 126 | 79 | 3 |
| Total† | 3,084 | 4,352 | 2,685 | 249 |

**Notes**
* This includes aggregate data from Transplant Québec to supplement national totals. Waiting list statistics for simultaneous kidney–pancreas (SKP) transplants are included in the pancreas section.
† The Total row includes intestines and other (non-SKP) combination organ transplants.
**Source**
Canadian Organ Replacement Register, 2020, Canadian Institute for Health Information.

## Types of Organ Donors

There are different types of organ donors and some are more common than others. The various types of organ donations have their own individual advantages and disadvantages. Some controversies may be connected to the types of donation linked with that procedure.

**Living donor:** This type of donation allows for transplantation while the donor is still alive and healthy; less complication is involved. It also reduces wait times associated with organ transplant (Mayo Clinic, 2021). There are different types of this donation.

a) **Directed:** This involves people who are related to each other. For example, biological parents, siblings and cousins. The donor may also be from unrelated persons with a connection to the recipient such as a spouse, friend or colleague. This is the commonest type and it is intentional; the donor identifies the recipient (Mayo Clinic, 2021).

b) **Non-Directed:** This involves a donor who decides to donate for altruistic reasons. Here, the donor is neither related to nor knows the identity of the recipient of the organ. However, the medical compatibility of the parties is examined prior to the procedure. In this case, the donor may decide not to meet the recipient or if the policy in place allows for the interaction they may meet (Mayo Clinic, 2021).

c) **Paired exchange:** This involves two donors – Donor A and Donor B who are not matched to their individual recipients – Recipient A and Recipient B – because of blood type compatibility. But matches with the other person's recipient whose donor, in turn, matches their own. Thus, a swap occurs where Donor A donates to Recipient B and Donor be to Recipient A. It is important to note that this type only occurs with a Kidney transplant (Mayo Clinic, 2021).

**Deceased donor:** This involves the donation of an organ after a person has been certified dead. It can either be a neurological brain death or cardio-circulatory death as determined by two medical persons (CIHI, 2014). In North America, attempts would have been made to save the life and if death results then confirmation of death and the documentation of the time of death would be recorded before organ donation can be considered (BC Transplant, 2021). The decision to donate can be made by the individual if prior instruction was given or the family (Organ donor, 2021). This option has longer wait times compared to the living donation.

**Pediatric donor:** This involves organ donation for children. The size of the organ is essential for success in this population (Donate life, 2021). The deceased donor option is common with this population; there has been an increase in the rate in recent years (Beckman, 2019).

## Table

| Type of donor | 2010 | 2011 | 2012 | 2013 | 2014 | 2015 | 2016 | 2017 | 2018 | 2019 |
|---|---|---|---|---|---|---|---|---|---|---|
| Deceased (NDD and DCD) | 466 | 515 | 541 | 553 | 591 | 649 | 760 | 803 | 761 | 820 |
| NDD | 424 | 456 | 459 | 489 | 470 | 511 | 588 | 604 | 538 | 580 |
| DCD | 42 | 59 | 82 | 64 | 121 | 138 | 172 | 199 | 223 | 240 |
| Living | 557 | 521 | 538 | 585 | 553 | 563 | 544 | 535 | 555 | 614 |

**Notes**
NDD: Neurological determination of death (donation after brain death).
DCD: Donation after cardio-circulatory death. 1 deceased donor in 2018 had missing data regarding donor type (NDD or DCD) and was excluded.
**Source**
Canadian Organ Replacement Register, 2020, Canadian Institute for Health Information.

## Ethical Consideration of Transplant Procedure
Organ transplant procedures are governed by ethical

considerations and conduct that must be adhered to. Some of the following address the areas of ethical consideration. These areas are also linked with some controversial debates.

**Consent:** Typically, there are various ways consent for an organ transplant is obtained and some are preferred over the other.

a) **Routine removal** – In this type, the state has the authority to remove organs from the deceased because they claim ownership of the body of the deceased. This is most common with Communist society and involves the opt-out model (Institute of Medicine, 2006).

b) **Presumed consent** – Individuals are given the right to refuse organ donation after death, this refusal will be officially documented. Thus, consent for organ donation is presumed if there is no documented proof of refusal; it also involves the opt-out policy model. This model can involve a strong policy – Families do not have to be consulted about organ donation or a weak policy – families must be consulted. In the strong policy model families are still consulted about the family / medical history even though it's not mandatory. Countries like Spain and Belgium use this model. (Institute of Medicine, 2006).

c) **Informed consent** – Donors or families of the donor give express consent about their willingness to donate an organ. This is the most preferred method and it is commonly used in the United States and Canada.

This involves the opt-in policy model (Institute of Medicine, 2006).

**Allocation parameters:** The allocation of organs is associated with ethical policy adherence. Some countries have a legal working policy while others may not have this, ethics should nevertheless be embedded in the decision-making process. In the United States, for example, the need for an independent governing entity was recognized as important. Thus, the Organ Procurement and Transplantation Network was born (OPTN) – this organization is responsible for the distribution of organs for transplantation in accordance with the legal policy; they are self-regulated by the transplant community (Van Meter, 1999).

To assist the OPTN in relevant matters the United Network for Organ Sharing (UNOS) was created. UNOS is a private not-for-profit organization overseen by the representatives of the transplant community and comprises of different stakeholders such as the donors, the recipients, family relatives of the donor, organizations – National Kidney Association; American Heart Association amongst others; transplant centres as well as organ procurement agencies (Van Meter, 1999).

According to OPTN and UNOS (2021), allocation procurement begins with screening all transplant candidates for medical compatibility with the donor and the incompatible matches are removed. A computerized process and ranked order of offer is then engaged – geography and right-sized organs play a role, the top-ranked are deemed to be those in urgent need. Other factors that are unique to each organ and associated with the organ allocation process are:

- Kidney – wait-time, pediatric status, distance from the hospital (donor's), survival benefit, prior living donor, Immune system incompatibility for donor and recipient.

- Liver – Medical Urgency, pediatric status and distance from the hospital (donor's)

- Lung – Medical Urgency, wait-time, survival benefit, distance from the hospital (donor's) and pediatric status

- Heart – Medical urgency, distance from the hospital (donor's) and pediatric status.

Preservation of organs is important for success. The peak organ preservation times are hearts and lungs 4-6 hours; liver 8-12 hours; pancreas 12-18 hours and kidney 24-36 hours.

## Controversies Surrounding Different Areas of Ethics Related to Organ Transplants

a)  **Consent:** There have been debates surrounding the issue of consent. Some argue that the presumed model would effectively increase the number of donors which could help keep many people alive; it is also debated that if the model was not successful it won't be in place nor would it be used. Further, it is reported that countries with the presumed consent opt-out model generally have more organ donation rates which can sometimes be 30% higher than the countries in the informed consent opt-in model. On the other hand, questions about how effectiveness is measured come into play, that is if the rate of organ donation is a good yardstick for measuring effectiveness and increase in the number of the Organ donor. Certainly, countries with successful opt-out models have incorporated other measures to make it impactful. There is no one way to determine the reason for the success of the opt-out models; it is a combination of factors (Institute of Medicine, 2006).

b) **Cost-effectiveness:** There are discussions around how cost-effective using a presumed consent model would be because to be ethical presumed consent model involves a thorough understanding of the process. For example, it would involve the education of the public which involves a rigorous process. The argument, therefore, is would it not be better for countries, for example, the United States, using the informed consent style to address whatever shortcomings the model has and make it effective than to switch to the presumed consent model which although touted to increase the rate of organ donors would involve a significant amount of money (Institute of Medicine, 2006).

c) **Autonomy:** The controversy here is with the informed consent model where except consent is expressly given it is assumed that the individual would not have been willing to donate organs. However, arguments around this are that most people express willingness to donate organs during the discussion which infers that consent can be presumed when deceased (Institute of Medicine, 2006).

## Allocation parameters:

As mentioned earlier for countries without firm legal policies around the allocation of organs ethical practices are still encouraged. For countries with a laid-out process of operation as described earlier controversies around the allocation process have been aired. A study by the C4 Article contributors in 2018 on the current opinion in organ allocation argued that the participation of the transplant community in the organ allocation policy may unduly influence the decision-making process.

Moreover, when the same institution governing the organ transplant process is also tasked with addressing the transplant community affairs then there's less productivity and policy advancement. Further, multiple involvements may lead to bias, obliterate justice and the public trust which will not portray the main goal of the policy. They proffered that there be better reporting from stakeholders and the institutions should be dynamic with a result-producing mindset.

The Authors also argued that not much importance is awarded to the patients' preferences. The policy does not take the patient's perspective into account although it was certainly created to safeguard them. Therefore, an approach that would incorporate this should be adopted and the policy updated to reflect it.

## Controversies Surrounding Different Organ Transplants

There are controversies that exist and are unique or common with a particular organ. These disagreements could be related to the type of donor process, ethical aspect of the transplant process or the general effectiveness of the transplant process in a particular organ.

a) **Kidney:** Paired exchange programs are a controversial topic in the kidney organ transplant community. These programs form a network of chains where kidney donor numbers increase from interconnected donors. These exchanges can sometimes be trans-country thus a program known as the Global Kidney Exchange (GKE) was created. This program aims to link donor and recipient pairs from different (wealthy and non-wealthy) countries. GKE works by connecting a person in a wealthy country whose donor is incompatible with a donor-recipient pair in a poor country who might match each other. The pair in the low-income country are unable to pay for the cost of treatment. GKE would settle the bill but the donors are often uncompensated for wages lost (Ro, 2021).

The controversy here is two-fold – 1. The pair in the low-income country were already matched and did not need the pair in the high-come country who were unmatched. What they required was medical funding, if they had this GKE program would not be unnecessary. 2. The organ transplant procedure takes place in the high-income country and upon completion, the pair from the high-income country would receive premium care while the pair from the poor country returns back to their country with little to no post-operative care. This disparity in the care received is the issue here.

Finally, the wealth imbalance between the pairs brings tomind the idea of organ trafficking. Thus, GKE is often viewed as a program that obtains organs from financially disadvantaged people. This practice would encourage more illegal organ sale from countries where such exist. Globally, People could also be under duress to donate kidneys (Ro, 2021).

b) **Lungs:** The effectiveness of lung transplant in persons with Chronic Obstructive Pulmonary Disease is debatable. This condition produces an inflation of the lungs and a shortage of oxygen; the treatment has been to encourage lifestyle modification such as smoking cessation and oxygen therapy. The speed of disease progression to respiratory failure, if any, differs per person hence there remains an ongoing argument about the right time to transplant. Some people argue that lung transplant in this population holds no true value (Trindade and Palmer, 2004).

## Controversies Surrounding Different Population Organ Transplants

**Pediatrics population:** In this population, the time at which an individual is certified as dead is an important and contentious issue. A study by the Committee on Bioethics (2013) on ethical controversies in organ donation after circulatory death addressed this point. A party argued that the period a person dies is essential if ethics must be maintained. It is not acceptable to directly take a person's life for the purpose of donation and the person must already be dead before any organ removal; ideally following the 2-5 minutes wait-time, to do otherwise is to be unethical.

However, another party debated that it is not unethical if a person or the family on behalf of a person elected to be taken off life-support. With this, the individual's organ can be collected if consent is obtained without necessarily adhering to the dead donor rule—a rule to certify the person as dead.

**Prisoners:** Prisoners who are in need of an organ transplant is a controversial topic. On one hand, people understand that it is their constitutional right to receive it if they are in line for it. However, the cost of receiving one is quite high considering the person's status and the fact others who are lawful citizens are still waiting—it is arguably the question of is this truly necessary? Conversely, UNOS declared that the lawful status of a person should not dictate when to receive a transplant. Another controversy is the issue of prisoners as organ donors; the appropriateness of this is questioned. Some believe that if another life can be saved with a prisoner's organs when he is on death row it is not inappropriate and not doing so is a waste. Others feel caution should be exercised to prevent organ donation compulsion (Prison legal news, 2014).

**Population with a religious and cultural view:** People of different religious beliefs may have a controversial view of organ transplants. Ethno-cultural factors can also play a role where people of certain cultures would rather not participate in organ donation. There is no explicit writing to decry organ donation in various religions. However, certain practices within each religion may explain why some people have a negative view of it. Regardless, of the religion or culture, the rate of organ donation decreases when religious or cultural attitudes towards the body of a deceased person and organ donations are not aligned (Eshraghian, 2013).

## Conclusion

The process of Organ transplants has grown over the years primarily to help improve the rate of organ donations across the globe. The process was built on the principle of Justice and Utility, therefore, despite its many controversies spanning across types of donation, ethics and population, the procedure has saved lives and improved the quality of life of individuals. There is certainly room for improvement in policy and policy administration but it is a constantly evolving field and in coming years further progress is anticipated.

# Chapter 9:

# The Modern Perceptions and Depictions of Organ Donation and Transplantation

By: Christina MacDonald and Suad Alad

## How Are Organ Transplants Viewed in the World Today?

Organ transplantation is widely seen as a great modern medical achievement. At an individual level, there may be various qualms about the major surgical procedures, but what is more often perpetuated are the emotional videos of organ transplant recipients meeting those who have donated or stories of the multiple lives saved by an organ donor after their death. For instance, in 2019, the news and lifestyle program *Good Morning America* reported the meeting of a 22-year-old liver donor with a 19-year-old transplant recipient (Kindelan, 2019). Depicted as a very emotional and heartwarming encounter, this is only one of many examples of how organ transplants are viewed as a very important and life-saving procedure amongst the general public.

Throughout this chapter, the modern view of organ donation and transplantation will be further explored by taking a deeper look into religious perspectives, how pop culture—specifically television (TV) and social media—can influence public perceptions, as well as use philosophical and sociological lenses to analyze current perceptions.

## Disclaimer

The perspectives discussed in this chapter may better represent the modern Western perception of organ transplants. The majority of accessible information on this topic is from Western sources and may not reflect perceptions in all parts of the world, especially areas in which there is less documented research or places in the world where medicinal practices differ. It must also be acknowledged that generalizations of views are just that, generalizations. Individuals can have differing views on organ transplantation in their own personal lives that may not be reflected by the larger generalized 'world' views that will be discussed objectively throughout this chapter.

## Nuances of Organ Donation
## (Quick Review for Chapter 8)

Organ donors can be living or deceased. Living donors undergo surgery to donate certain organs, such as a piece of their liver or one of their kidneys—the liver is able to regenerate and only one kidney is required for adequate bodily function (Michalopoulos, 2007; National Kidney Foundation, 2015). Registered donors, once deceased, give all possibly viable organs to be used for transplantation. Moreover, depending on the country one lives in, the process of organ donation after death differs.

The two prominent systems for organ donation after death are the opt-in (expressive consent) and opt-out (presumed consent) system. The difference is that opt-in requires the future donor to register to be a donor whereas opt-out automatically registers people as future donors, and the individual must register their objection if they do not want to donate (Zink et al., 2005). Regarding living donors, Iran is an outlier in their organ transplant process because, instead of having a donation process they have a legal and regulated organ trade—organs are bought and sold, not donated (Major, 2008).

## Views on the Medical Procedure of Organ Transplants

Although the recipient of an organ transplant may feel immense relief and gratitude, the process of transplantation is not a simple procedure. The process of organ transplantation, as discussed in more detail in Chapter 5, involves surgery—which is invasive and can have complications— after-surgery procedures and check-ins, a lengthy recovery process, anti-rejection medication and can impact one's emotional well-being (HRSA, n.d.). Even so, those who are able to undergo organ transplantation are often considered to be extremely fortunate as the process to get on a waiting list and then receive an organ can take years. As of February 2021, over 107,000 people in the United States were on the transplant waiting list (HRSA, 2021). Considering there were around 39, 000 transplants performed in the United States in 2020, there is a high demand, but low supply of life-saving transplants underway (HRSA, 2021). Looking at these statistics alone, it is understandable why those who undergo transplant surgery are perceived as fortunate, relative to their circumstances.

A living donor's experience after surgery will range as people have different recovery rates, but generally, they can expect to feel more fatigued and will need to monitor their activity levels. Moreover, donors will have to be more cautious and understand that their lifestyles must be cognizant of the higher risks associated with their donation, for example, donating one kidney will result in the need to be more protective of the one kidney they have left (National Kidney Foundation, 2019). The majority of donors report positive feelings after donating, however, the varying psychological impacts of this body-altering surgery cannot be neglected (National Kidney Foundation, 2019).

The process is viewed as life-saving, but it is not guaranteed to be free of complications for the recipient or the donor. Experiences before, during, and after surgery are subjective and unique, but the general perception of the process is that it is extremely valuable and often saves and improves the quality of life of the recipient.

## Religion and Organ Donation and Transplantation

There may be a widespread impression that organ donation and transplantation would not be accepted in many religions due to other practices that aim to preserve bodies quickly after death, or that do not allow for certain medical procedures. For example, Jewish customs honour the deceased by burying them soon after death, ideally within the same day. Even if there is a slight postponement due to various exceptions, it should occur as quickly as possible (Klug, n.d.). Similarly, in Islam, it is customary that one should also be buried soon after death, often no longer than 24 hours after passing (Rahman, 2011). Moreover, Jehovah's Witnesses have short funeral ceremonies that are not required to be conducted quickly, usually being held within a week of death (Paul Williams Independent Funeral Directors Ltd., n.d.). What they are known for is their refusal to undergo blood transfusions (Boggi et al., 2004).

Even with these practices, these religions, as well as most other major religions—including Amish, Baptist, Catholicism, many other Christian denominations, Buddhism, and Hinduism—allow for or do not have a stance on organ transplants (National Kidney Foundation, 2017). What can be seen throughout the religions that allow for donation and transplantation is that these acts are seen as life-saving and acts of charity. Some religions may leave the decision completely to the individual, while others believe acts of donation and transplantation to be acceptable when it is very certain that it will aid in improving the health of the recipient (National Kidney Foundation, 2017). Although formally, many religions are not opposed to organ donation and transplants, there may be cultural or personal forces at play in people's lives that make them opposed to this procedure.

It should be noted that Jehovah's Witnesses provide a unique perspective on organ donation and transplants due to the fact that blood transfusions are refused. At first, it may not seem like an organ transplant can occur without blood transfer, but Jehovah's Witnesses accept solid organs (Boggi et al., 2004). Solid organs —which includes the kidneys and pancreas— are able to be transplanted without transfusion. There may be complications and later medical issues that can cause medical and ethical issues surrounding this, however, when looking on the surface level at the procedure of transplantation, when organs and tissues are drained of blood, the donation procedure is allowed (Boggi et al., 2004; National Kidney Foundation, 2017).

## How Popular Culture Can Educate Society on Organ Donation and Transplantation

With the modern world becoming one and the same with a techno-social one (a society or community whose social and institutional practices are interconnected with their relationships with technology) (Chayko, 2016), perceptions, deceptions and influences regarding a wide spread of topics become vehemently more accessible to the general public, regardless of age, race, sexual orientation, gender or class. On the surface, this appears to be a wonderful educational advancement that otherwise would require extensive pre-existing knowledge in order to engage with such conversations. In the rise of mass media consumption, someone can learn just as much from an academic setting as they would from a fiction-based film influenced by real-world events, a thread posted to Twitter.com with educational intention, or from a video clip or essay posted on Youtube.com with a similar educational objective because this form of education is continuing and presents tangible concepts within a contemporary setting (Lynch, 2020). With this information in mind, it appears as though the media is adapting, and seemingly for the better. In relation to organ donation and transplantation, this form of influence and education is highly applicable. Before delving into the topic further, an understanding of television and other forms of mass media's ability to educate a vast group of individuals needs to be acknowledged and dissected.

In the past two decades, there has been a surge of medical dramas within TV entertainment. Medical dramas are fictional pieces of media that follow the personal and professional lives of those who work in the medicinal field. Although they have existed for the last six decades, since the release of popular medical drama *Grey's Anatomy* (2005-Present, Rhimes), they have become much more common on TV—with other successful releases such as *The Good Doctor* (US) (Kim & Shore, 2017-Present), *House M.D.* (Shore, 2004-2012), *Chicago Med* (Olmstead & Wolf, 2015-Present) and *New Amsterdam* (Schulner, 2018-Present). Although different in character dynamic, plot, and production, each show plays a significant role in the exposure of medicinal, surgical, pharmaceutical and psychiatric practices beyond what is described or addressed in mundane interactions, such as googling symptoms. It also provides a more intimate form of medical exposure that regulated medical check-ups conducted within day to day life would not provide.

With this in mind, it is no surprise that when seeking a more informal approach towards education, those not typically surrounded by or exposed to medical discourse or knowledge turn to the televised medical dramas for exposure. Yes, these stories are fictional, and those who are consuming this form of media are aware of that, however, there is only so much of it that can be fictional or 'untrue' as the illnesses, the practices and the professions are a reality for many.

In his 1964 novel, *Understanding Media: The Extensions of Man*, Canadian Philosopher Marshall McLuhan claims that real-life medical interns who observe medical procedures feel as though their experience mimics a first-person perspective and interaction, rather than an outside view and that they gain more knowledge through this first-hand observation because the interaction is so intimate (McLuhan, 1964). In his thirty-first chapter *Television: The Timed Giant* McLuhan writes that this form of intimacy is applicable to televised media and that it allows the audience a chance to experience what is being presented on their screens first-hand rather than watching something happening in the background. This, by extension, suggests that those watching medical dramas are learning more about medical procedures and the medicinal field as a whole, whether or not that is their intention when watching each series.

It is important to recognize that this informal education is not a replacement for academia or educational institutions. In saying that, it is also important to recognize *who* is being educated by this method of unorthodox teachings and whether or not these teachings are affecting these same individuals who make up this viewership.

## How Do the Portrayals of Organ Donation and Transplantation in Mass/Social Media Negatively Affect the Real World?

As previously stated, the potential to learn from TV is present and should be recognized as a contemporary educational outlet. There is no doubt that this access to education, regardless of primary exposure to academia, has positive effects. However, complications arise when those writing about these shows have a primary goal to entertain *before* educating, even if the topics being used for entertainment reflect and engage with real-world concepts and events. A short interview titled *The Purpose of Education* (2012), with American philosopher and linguist Noam Chomsky illustrates that with shifting technologies of education (in this instance, entertainment media and TV) there needs to be a primary interest or desire to learn. If for whatever reason, this desire or motivation is not possessed, the information being presented is not observed with an educational lens and it essentially appears as "factoids that don't mean anything" (Youtube, 2012). He also states that the potential for a proper, well-rounded education also appears to fall flat if there is a lack of critical thought. If at any time the information being presented seems inaccurate, one should actively proceed with caution.

So, how does this lead to the education of organ donation and transplantation? Who is learning from these shows? Are these entertaining methods of education responsible, accurate and helpful? Do they provide crucial information to those who would otherwise not have formal exposure to medical information teachings? The answer to these questions, unfortunately, is a bit complicated.

A study conducted by the Department of General Surgery and Organ Transplantation in the Bozyaka Teaching Hospital found that the individuals affected the most by mass media representation of organ donation and transplantation are non-white citizens, elderly citizens, and citizens who fit within the categories of both these subgroups (Aykas et al., 2015). The study found that out of any form of widespread programming, TV and mass media was a primary source of education and basic information regarding organ donation. While TV shows and films about the medicinal field delve into information that is applicable to the real world, the objective of these productions is not necessarily to educate their audiences but to entertain them. Since it is not the audiences' responsibility to fact check, they may blindly trust that what they are consuming on TV is in fact accurate and true. Unfortunately, this is not always the case.

In 1980, the popular BBC show *Panorama* (1953-Present), aired an episode which claimed that 2 in every 100 people are pronounced brain dead when they have promising potential for recovery and that, essentially, their organs are immorally harvested for donation prematurely. Despite this being untrue, organ donation rates dropped significantly and it took 15 months for these referral rates to return to their normal position (Aykas et al., 2015). In the same study, it was found that traditional new outlets similarly had a negative influence on the understanding of organ donation and transplantation and, despite being methods of media that relied heavily on factual accuracy, they too fall victim to the same issues entertainment media have (Aykas et al., 2015).

In 2012, a Swiss mentor of public health accused doctors in Germany were desperate for organs and resuscitated a patient who was already proclaimed as dead in order to harvest them. This claim increased negative opinions regarding organ donation and the refusal rate dropped 53% (Aykas et al., 2015).

A similar article published in the 19th volume of *Clinical Transportation* found that while professionals involved in the process of organ donation and transplantation easily wrote off inaccurate or negative portrayals of organ donation as "only Hollywood", their studies concluded that because what was being presented on TV were encounters that could happen in the real world, it affected decisions regarding consensual organ donations (Morgan et al., 2005). This feeling of hesitancy only intensified as on-screen portrayals of failed procedures were highlighted throughout the shows they discussed seeing.

## How Social/Mass Media Positively Influences and Impacts Organ Donation and Transplantation

With this information in mind, it's important to recognize the incredible presence of mass media and how its influence within the general public is extremely prevalent, especially in today's world. Whether it be through TV or film, or regular news outlets, the media plays a large role in decisions people make regarding their health and everyday lives; especially if what is being presented to them is negative.

What does this mean if the presentation of medical procedures or information is shown in a positive light? Do the feelings of those influenced by the negative possibilities change? Or does the negative information pertain to them more clearly and appear factually accurate?

It is extremely clear that the presentation of medial influence impacts the decisions made by everyday citizens and that this is vehemently true when the representation is negative. However, this is not the only form of influence media has on the general public; there is also an argument for positive portrayals in televised media. Referring back to the Bozyaka Teaching Hospital, researchers found that when presentations and on-screen portrayals of organ donation was positive, it made the audiences watching each show feel more at ease and more inclined to consider donation if they were not already signed up or in the process of signing up (Aykas et al., 2015). In a sample survey conducted with 4500 individuals, it was found that regularly viewing popular medical dramas such as *Grey's Anatomy* (2005-Present, Rhimes) helped them better understand the importance of becoming donors and that of those 4500, 10% genuinely considered becoming donors in the future.

Similarly, a study published in *Proceedings of the National Academy of Sciences* found that the way in which organ donation is described within the series plays a crucial role in influencing peoples' feelings toward the whole process. Typically storylines that appeared to follow a more personal route (donating to family or loved ones) made people feel emotionally involved, making them more likely to consider donating (Harel et al., 2017). In relation to positive portrayals of organ donation and transplantation, media coverage beyond fictional branches was found to be just as persuasive and influential. Influence is based on whether the story regarding the person who is either in need of the transplant or the person donating the organs are presented positively or not. The study found that if the person seeking the donation were perceived within a negative light, blame-shifting was much more common and consideration of organ donation decreased drastically (Harel et al., 2017). However, it was found this presentation was not as likely, and that most donation stories were positive from beginning to end.

Continuing with the social aspects of organ donation and transplantation, social media can be used as a good outlet for information as well as gaining access to these resources. With the rise of social media and its inevitable incorporation into the medical field, surgeons have found that social media allows them to provide patient education in an accessible way (Henderson et al., 2019). Social media has also improved the standards of patient delivery, quality and care and has leveraged programs for patients to find living donors within their area and to "promote access to living donor education in culturally sensitive ways for [marginalized] populations" (Henderson et al., 2019).

Of the 299 members of the American Society of Transplant Surgeons (ASTS) that were surveyed regarding social media influence, 55% agreed that the use of social media facilitation should be used within seeking donor options for patients, as long as an additional screening is conducted. Furthermore, many were in agreement that the use of social media interaction can begin to delegitimize inaccurate deceptions of organ donation and "encompasses multifaceted communication tools" in the education and awareness of organ donation (Henderson et al., 2019).

## Looking Through a Sociological Lens:
## Post-Structuralism

After analyzing how the different forms of media can influence perceptions, an interesting lens to consider falls within the study of sociology. Sociology methodically looks at groups of humans and how they interact. In recognizing the dynamic relations of people with each other, as well as with larger social systems, the study of sociology is able to distinguish the social implications of people's everyday thoughts and actions (Ravelli & Webber, 2019). There are many different theories that take various approaches to analyzing social behaviours, norms, and structures, but one lens of interest when looking into the modern perception of organ transplants is post-structuralism.

Post-structuralist theory is a contemporary sociological theory that focuses on the social production of knowledge. In this theory, there is an understanding of the influence of power relations on what is understood as the 'truth' in society (Ravelli & Webber, 2019).

## Looking Into the Post-Structuralist Work
## of Michel Foucault

Michel Foucault was a French philosopher whose contributions to sociology fall under the lens of post-structuralist theory. Foucault is recognized for looking at the dynamic and intersecting relationship of power and knowledge (Ravelli & Webber, 2019). To connect this to organ transplantation, those who are disseminating the widespread knowledge about the necessity of organ donation and organ transplants are bodies in power (i.e. medical institutions and the government). This will be explored in further depth in the following section.

In his work, Foucault uses the term discourse as a "system of meaning that governs how we think, act, and speak about a particular thing or issue" (Ravelli & Webber, 2019). This is an important concept to understand when looking to analyze the modern perception of organ transplants as the language used surrounding the topic can influence how the majority view it. Looking at language use from a psychological standpoint, it can have great impacts on emotion as humans are able to give arbitrary letter and sound combinations abstract meanings (Lindquist, 2015). The use of specific language in discourse can play a powerful role in influencing one's perceptions as it can target human emotion.

## Discourse in Mass Media, the Government and Religion

Using Foucault's idea of discourse and the understanding that language plays a great role in influencing people's perception, there are some commonalities in how the media, governments and religions speak about organ donation and transplantations. Returning to the *Good Morning America* example discussed at the beginning of this chapter, the reporter covering the story often uses the words "guardian angel" to describe the organ donor. Within TV, as previously stated, stories or narratives that are emotionally invested in the positive outcomes of organ donations are typically the ones used to encourage donation in the first place. When the on-screen portrayal show's narratives revolving around family or marital donations, or donations where the donor died tragically, but their family decides to donate their organs because the character "just wanted to help others", emotional influence is used in order to describe the act of donation as selfless and rewarding (Morgan et al., 2005).

On sites speaking about religious standpoints on organ donation and transplantation, phrases such as "act of neighbourly love", "act of charity", "better human life", and "expression of sacrificial love" (National Kidney Foundation, 2017) are used as encouragement as well. Moreover, organ donation information websites, as well as government websites use similar language with phrases such as "Sign Up to Save Lives: Be An Organ Donor", "Can I really make a difference?", and "The Chance to Give" (Gift of Life Donor Program, n.d.; HRSA, 2021). This form of persuasive language is even found in methods of academic writing such as journal articles. An article written by Moritsugu (2013), is entitled *The power of organ donation to save lives through transplantation.* The point of highlighting the consistent use of words and phrases that carry a sense of honour, public service and heroism is not to say that these messages are untruthful, but rather to reveal that the discourse created by the large platforms that govern how society views organ transplantation and donation is highly influential.

However, it is important to remember that while society has standards of care that human beings should extend to one another, caring for oneself and one's right to bodily autonomy are extremely important. Helping others in whatever way one can is a gratuitous thing to do, and organ donation is just one of the many ways to be gratuitous.

## Conclusion

The exposure and awareness of organ donation and transplantation are adapting along with the adaptation of media and its educational and influential promise. Perceptions regarding its procedures, processes, impacts and social implications are expected to change as society progresses forward. Accessibility of information regarding organ donation and transplantation must be at the forefront, allowing individuals to better understand the implications of the procedure from multiple standpoints—societal, religious, personal, to name a few. Only with accessibility may an accurate, universal, and modern perception inclusive of multiple perspectives and accurate in its presentation of information regarding this life-changing procedure.

# Chapter 10:

# The Future of Organ Transplantations

By: Sriraam Sivachandran

**Organ Transplantations**

In many cases, patients suffer from certain diseases that cause permanent damage to various vital organs. The organs then become non-functional, making them essentially useless. There are certain organs that can be transplanted in order to save a patient's life. The most commonly transplanted organs are the kidney, liver, heart, pancreas, lung, and small intestine (CDC, 2019). Majority of organs that are donated come from deceased donors, but some organs, such as the kidney, lungs, and liver, can be donated from living donors as they are most likely only donating a part of the specific organ.

Even though someone may need an organ and there are available organs that have been donated, there are still some criteria that must be met in order to match donors and recipients. Examples of important criteria are blood type, body size, and severity of patient's condition (Health Resources & Services Administration, 2018). The issue that still remains with organ transplantation is the fact that there are many patients that are put on a waiting list because the number of recipients outnumbers the amount of available donations. The United States Department of Health and Human Services and the Health Resources & Services Administration have specific statistics that outline the root of the problem. As discussed in chapter 9, as of February 2021, there are over 107,000 people that are on the United States national waiting list and this includes men, women and children (Health Resources & Services Administration, 2021a). In the United States, the kidney is one of the most requested organs. Specifically, in 2020 over 80,000 people were on the waiting list for a kidney, but approximately only 20,000 people actually received their kidney transplant (Health Resources & Services Administration, 2021a). Seeing as though there are still many people on organ transplantation waiting lists, it comes into question whether there will be any improvement in the current process. How sustainable is the current organ transplantation pathway and how many more people will die by being on the waiting list and not actually get a new organ?

With the advancement of technology and the development of novel scientific methods, it is plausible that there are current advancements in the process of organ transplantation. There are certain methods that are being used today that attempt to find a more effective way of presenting end-stage organ failure patients an alternative solution to the regular organ transplantation process. Even though these methods are still trying to be understood, their emergence and current research is a step in the right direction as it broadens the scientific and medical communities to new avenues of organ transplantation that may eventually become the norm.

## Whole-Organ Bioengineering

As the number of organ recipients continue to pile up while the number of organ donations continues to plateau, there has been a glaring problem of organ shortage. In order to combat this major problem, scientists have attempted to use the method of tissue engineering. Simply, the main goal of tissue engineering is to create tissues or whole organs that have the same capabilities as regular organs in order for them to be used as replacement organs in patients that suffer from end-stage organ failure (Peloso et al., 2015).

There have been many different hypotheses and technologies that arose because of the originality of tissue engineering, but the most promising technology that was developed was whole organ decellularization. Whole organ decellularization would be used to create a three-dimensional extracellular matrix of a specific tissue and it would allow that extracellular matrix to have the same structure and characteristics as the original tissue (Peloso et al., 2015). In order to decellularize a specific tissue of an organ, the organ has to be cleared with specific detergents that eliminate all the cell components except for the extracellular matrix components and molecules (Crapo et al., 2011). There are different detergents that have been used in different tissue decellularization projects. However, the whole process of decellularization depends on certain tissue factors such as tissue density, thickness and cellularity (Peloso et al., 2015). There are also specific reasons as to why the extracellular matrix is an important part of the whole tissue decellularization process.

Firstly, the extracellular matrix allows cells to communicate with surrounding cells and the tissue environment because it is in equilibrium with the surrounding tissue (Peloso et al., 2015). The extracellular matrix also allows for organ specific properties that include physical, biochemical, and biomechanical properties (Peloso et al., 2015). While the functions of all three of these vary, they are only able to perform their functions because of the extracellular matrix. Lastly, the extracellular matrix contributes to cell attachment and tissue integration and development because of certain growth and bio-inductive factors that are contained within it (Peloso et al., 2015).

There are three summarized steps that explain the whole process of tissue decellularization. As explained previously, the first step involves the use of various ionic (positive charge) and anionic (negative charge) detergents that clear the original cells and the only component that is left is the extracellular matrix framework and structure. This step is deemed as the decellularization process (Peloso et al., 2015). The end product of the first step is the three-dimensional extracellular matrix framework that has the original tissue's framework. The second step is more of an analysis phase which allows for the framework to be analyzed (Peloso et al., 2015). The analysis of the framework allows researchers to check for certain criteria. For example, they would be able to see whether the original tissue's structure is actually preserved in the extracellular matrix framework. They are also able to see whether important growth factors are contained within the extracellular matrix and they can also analyse the framework's biological properties. The last step of the whole decellularization process is inserting organ-specific cells into the framework (Peloso et al., 2015). One of the most important aspects of the last step to understand is that in order to avoid any future medical problems, the inserted cells should really come from the patient that will actually receive the biologically engineered organ. This step is deemed as the recellularization process (Peloso et al., 2015). Unfortunately, there are certain complications that come about with the recellularization step. First of all, a large number of cells need to be used in order to make up the whole three-dimensional extracellular matrix framework. Researchers also have to make sure there are certain proportions of cells that have to be met in order for the biologically engineered organ to be functional and to make sure that the cells actually develop once they are in the extracellular matrix framework (Peloso et al., 2015).

## Xenotransplantation

Another future option that has been gaining steam in the medical community is xenotransplantation. Xenotransplantation has been a polarizing solution that has been proposed to aid in the shortage of organ donations. This process involves the organs of one species being transplanted into another different species; which in this case would be an animal to a human (Altinörs, 2020). The idea of xenotransplantation had been discussed in the past, but due to advancements in the medical community, researchers are able to see whether it may be a more viable option in the future. Currently, there are studies being conducted that test whether heart, kidney, liver, and lung xenotransplantation can occur successfully in different models (Ekser et al., 2017). Majority of the studies that are currently being conducted are attempting to complete successful transplantation from a specific animal into a non-human primate. For example, a study conducted by Cooper et al in 2017 showed that there was successful transplantation of pig liver xenografts into non-human primates and they survived between seven to nine days (Cooper et al., 2017).

Even though there has been increased xenotransplantation between animals and there is the potential for xenotransplantation between animals and humans, there are many obstacles that researchers have to overcome before xenotransplantation can be widely accepted. Firstly, there are certain immunological barriers that may pose great danger to the whole process of xenotransplantation. The main immunological barriers that researchers must be aware of is organ rejection (Vanderpool, 1999). Furthermore, one of the more prominent issues that come along with xenotransplantation is the ethical conundrum (Vanderpool, 1999). There are many ethical questions that people against xenotransplantation may propose. Is the use and genetic modification of animals something that scientists should really be focusing on? Who will be the first human subjects in the test clinical trials? How will the idea of xenotransplantation be broached and explained to the general public? Even if researchers were eventually able to successfully complete xenotransplantation between animals and humans, there will still be some major obstacles that must be overcome before the idea of xenotransplantation is accepted past the medical community.

## Nuclear Reprogramming

Stem cell research is an area of focus that has been well researched over the past years due to the multitude of application possibilities. Researchers have observed that the expression of certain genes in mature cells can give rise to induced pluripotent stem cells (Platt & Cascalho, 2013). The expression of the genes from the mature cells can be considered the first step of how we can gain access to these induced pluripotent stem cells. In order for the mature cells to express those specific genes, the transfer of viral transforming genes must be done first (Platt & Cascalho, 2013). The positive component of these induced pluripotent stem cells is that they have cloning factors. This is an important aspect of this future method because the reprogrammed cells that will eventually be put in the recipient would be generated from themselves (Platt & Cascalho, 2013). The drawback of nuclear reprogramming of cell is that although the induced pluripotent stem cells are able to create and reprogram certain cells because of their cloning factors, there is no clear inanimate organ that is being placed in the recipient (Platt & Cascalho, 2013). Simply, the problem that arises is that the cloned cells would be there without an actual organ to take the place of the non-function organ in the patient. Researchers have come up with some potential solutions that may help with this problem. One potential solution would be to simply implant the undifferentiated fetal cell into the patient and let in-vivo organ formation occur (Platt & Cascalho, 2013). This has been successful when using fetal cells but there has been no research into whether induced pluripotent stem cells can undergo in-vivo organ formation (Platt & Cascalho, 2013). If researchers are able to solve this problem and provide a viable long-term solution, induced pluripotent stem cells may be a practical alternative to whole organ transplantation.

## Organ Preservation

An important aspect of the whole organ transplantation process is what actually occurs before the organ is transplanted into the patient. In other words, how the organ is preserved before it reaches its final stage. As of right now, the most commonly used method to preserve donated organs is static cold storage. The process of static cold storage has been used since the 1960s (Jing et al., 2018). Donated organs that are in static cold storage are flushed with a specific solution that specialize in preservation (Jing et al., 2018). The temperature of the preservation solution must be between zero to four degrees Celsius. Next, the donated organ is submerged in the preservation solution until the transplantation actually takes place (Jing et al., 2018). The main reason as to why the donated organ stays in this cold preservation solution is because the cold environment is what actually decreases cellular metabolism and it provides protection against any harmful substances (Jing et al., 2018). Even though static cold storage is the main method being used today to preserve organs, there are still various limitations that decreases the effectiveness and usefulness of this method. For example, if the donated organ is submerged and placed in the cold preservation environment for too long, tissue damage may start to occur (Jing et al., 2018). Another downfall to static cold storage is that the longer the donated organ is in the cold preservation environment, the harder it is for doctors to assess the function and viability and there will be a decreasing chance of repairing the donated organ (Jing et al., 2018).

A proposed method that is currently being researched is the use of ex vivo machine perfusion and normothermic machine perfusion (Jing et al., 2018). Ex vivo machine perfusion can be thought of as repairing or reconditioning the donated organ before transplantation can occur (Jing et al., 2018). The main reason as to why this strategy has been gaining more attention is because it decreases the risk of any ischemia reperfusion injury. If ischemia reperfusion injury does occur, there is a greater chance that the donated organ will be dysfunctional at the early stages after transplantation and the chances of long term survival decreases greatly (Jing et al., 2018). There are several reasons that explain why ischemia reperfusion injury can occur in donated organs. These reasons include but are not limited to inflammation, vascular leakage, energy deficiency, and cell death (Jing et al., 2018). Therefore, the use of ex vivo machine perfusion can allow doctors and researchers to repair or recondition the donated organ in order for it to eliminate the possibility of undergoing any of those detrimental effects listed above.

On the other hand, normothermic machine perfusion is another strategy that is being researched to replace static cold storage (Jing et al., 2018). This method requires the donated organ to be placed under regular physiological conditions. Normothermic machine perfusion allows the donated organ to be under normal body temperature and is provided necessary substrates and oxygen (Jing et al., 2018). There are several advantages to the use of normothermic machine perfusion. As stated before, this method allows for the supplying of oxygen and nutrients to the donated organ and there is the capability to remove metabolic waste (Jing et al., 2018). If this method is used, doctors and researchers are still able to assess the donated organ and can conduct any required repairs that must be done (Jing et al., 2018). Lastly, one of the most important advantages is the decreased risk of ischemia reperfusion injury (Jing et al., 2018). By decreasing the chance of undergoing ischemia reperfusion injury, the donated organ has a greater probability for long term survival.

It is important to find future efficient strategies that also help with the preservation of organs as that may aid in the fight against the shortage of donated organs.

## Conclusion

Organ transplantation is an important medical procedure that has saved many people's lives. However, there has been an increased number of people that require organ transplants, while there has been a decreased number of donated organs. With the rising problem of organ shortage, the future of organ transplantation must be questioned, and alternatives must be found. Whole organ bioengineering, xenotransplantation, and nuclear programming are specific alternatives that are currently being researched. If there are any successful trials for any one of these alternatives, the future of organ transplantation is extremely encouraging.

# References

**Chapter 1:**

Aida, L. (2014). Alexis Carrel (1873–1944): Visionary vascular surgeon and pioneer in organ transplantation. Journal of Medical Biography, 22(3), 172-175. doi:10.1177/0967772013516899

Barker, C. F., & Markmann, J. F. (2013). Historical Overview of Transplantation. Cold Spring Harbor Perspectives in Medicine, 3(4). doi:10.1101/cshperspect.a014977

Brink J. G., Hassoulas J. (2009). The first human heart transplant and further advances in cardiac transplantation at Groote Schuur Hospital and the University of Cape Town. Cardiovasc J Afr. 20(1):31-35. https://www.ncbi.nlm.nih.gov/pmc/articles/ PMC4200566/

Cooper, D. K. (2018). Christiaan Barnard—The surgeon who dared: The story of the first human-to-human heart transplant. Global Cardiology Science and Practice, 2018(2). doi:10.21542/ gcsp.2018.11

HealthLinkBC (n.d.). Organ transplant. Retrieved from https://www.healthlinkbc.ca/health-topics/ty7522

Health Resources & Services Administration. (2018, December 04). Timeline of Historical Events and Significant Milestones. Retrieved from https://www.organdonor.gov/about/facts-terms/history.html

Hatzinger, M., Stastny, M., Grützmacher, P., & Sohn, M. (2016). Die Geschichte der Nierentransplantation. Der Urologe, 55(10), 1353-1359. doi:10.1007/s00120-016-0205-3

Júnior, R. F., Salvalaggio, P., Rezende, M. B., Evangelista, A. S., Guardia, B. D., Matielo, C. E., . . . Filho, S. P. (2015). Liver transplantation: History, outcomes and perspectives. Einstein (São Paulo), 13(1), 149-152. doi:10.1590/s1679-45082015rw3164

Mayo Clinic. (2021, April 27). Kidney transplant. Retrieved from https://www.mayoclinic.org/tests-procedures/kidney-transplant/about/pac-20384777

Nobel Lecture. (n.d.). The Nobel Prize in Physiology or Medicine 1912. Retrieved from https://www.nobelprize.org/prizes/medicine/1912/carrel/lecture/

SAMU P. C. (1960). Tissue transplantation and the homograft reaction. University of Toronto medical journal, 38, 39–51.

Setchell, B. P. (1990). The testis and tissue transplantation: Historical aspects. Journal of Reproductive Immunology, 18(1), 1-8. doi:10.1016/0165-0378(90)90020-7

Shayan, H. (2001). Organ Transplantation: From Myth to Reality. Journal of Investigative Surgery, 14(3), 135-138. doi:10.1080/089419301300343282

Singh, M., Nuutila, K., Collins, K., & Huang, A. (2017). Evolution of skin grafting for treatment of burns: Reverdin pinch grafting to Tanner mesh grafting and beyond. Burns, 43(6), 1149-1154. doi:10.1016/j.burns.2017.01.015

The Churchill Project. (2019, August 16). Sir Richard Molyneux and Churchill's Skin Graft. Retrieved from https://winstonchurchill.hillsdale.edu/sir-richard-molyneux-and-churchills-skin-graft/

United Network for Organ Sharing. (2018, May 22). History of Living Donation. Retrieved from https://transplantliving.org/living-donation/history/

U.S. Department of Veterans Affairs (2018, August 24). First Successful Liver Transplant, Retrieved from https://www.research.va.gov/research_in_action/First-successful-liver-transplant.cfm

Venuta, F., & Raemdonck, D. V. (2017). History of lung transplantation. Journal of Thoracic Disease, 9(12), 5458-5471. doi:10.21037/jtd.2017.11.84

What is Dialysis? (2021, March 23). Retrieved from https://www.kidney.org/atoz/content/dialysisinfo

Ziegler, U. E., Dietz, U. A., & Schmidt, K. (2004). Skin Grafts. Surgery in Wounds, 179-186. doi:10.1007/978-3-642-59307-9_18

**Chapter 2:**

Anderson, D., Billingham, R. E., Lampkin, G., & Medawar, P. B. (1951). The use of skin grafting to distinguish between monozygotic and dizygotic twins in cattle. Heredity, 5(3), 379-397. https://doi.org/10.1038/hdy.1951.38

Androutsos, G., Diamantis, A., & Vladimiros, L. (2008). The first leg transplant for the treatment of cancer by Saints Cosmas and Damian. Journal of B.U.ON. : official journal of the Balkan Union of Oncology, 13(2), 297–304.

Barker, C. F., & Markmann, J. F. (2013). Historical overview of transplantation. Cold Spring Harbor perspectives in medicine, 3(4), a014977. https://doi.org/10.1101/cshperspect.a014977

Brent L. (1997). The discovery of immunologic tolerance. Human immunology, 52(2), 75–81. https://doi.org/10.1016/S0198-8859(96)00289-3

British Society for Immunology. (2017). Transplant Immunology. Immunology.org. https://www.immunology.org/policy-and-public-affairs/briefings-and-position-statements/transplant-immunology.

Cinqualbre, J., & Kahan, B. D. (2002). René Küss: fifty years of retroperitoneal placement of renal transplants. Transplantation proceedings, 34(8), 3019–3025. https://doi.org/10.1016/s0041-1345(02)03626-6

Cooley D. A. (2002). America's First Nobel Prize in Medicine or Physiology: The Story of Guthrie and Carrel. Texas Heart Institute Journal, 29(2), 150–152.

Eghtesad, B., & Fung, J. (2017). Thomas Earl Starzl, MD, PhD (1926–2017): Father of Transplantation. International Journal of Organ Transplantation Medicine, 8(2), e1.

Hurst J. (2012). A modern Cosmas and Damian: Sir Roy Calne and Thomas Starzl receive the 2012 Lasker~Debakey Clinical Medical Research Award. The Journal of clinical investigation, 122(10), 3378–3382. https://doi.org/10.1172/jci66465

Redman, E. (2015). To Save His Dying Sister-In-Law, Charles Lindbergh Invented a Medical Device. Smithsonian Magazine. Retrieved from https://www.smithsonianmag.com/smithsonian-institution/save-his-dying-sister-law-charles-lindbergh-Invented-medical-device-180956526/.

Simpson E. (2015). Medawar's legacy to cellular immunology and clinical transplantation: a commentary on Billingham, Brent and Medawar (1956) 'Quantitative studies on tissue transplantation immunity. III. Actively acquired tolerance'. Philosophical transactions of the Royal Society of London. Series B, Biological sciences, 370(1666), 20140382. https://doi.org/10.1098/rstb.2014.0382

Southard, J. H., & Belzer, F. O. (1995). Organ preservation.
Annual review of medicine, 46, 235–247. https://doi.org/
10.1146/annurev.med.46.1.235

United Network for Organ Sharing. (2021). History of UNOS.
unos.org. https://unos.org/about/history-of-unos/.

Vernon G. (2019). Alexis Carrel: 'father of transplant surgery'
and supporter of eugenics. The British journal of general
practice : the journal of the Royal College of General
Practitioners, 69(684), 352. https://doi.org/10.3399/
bjgp19X704441

Wijdicks E. (2018). How Harvard Defined Irreversible Coma.
Neurocritical care, 29(1), 136–141. https://doi.org/10.1007/
s12028-018-0579-8

**Chapter 3:**
Baan, C. C. (2018). In Case you Missed It—Basic Science
Advances in Transplantation 2017. Transplantation, 102(6), 932–
934. doi: 10.1097/TP.0000000000002161.

Bezinover, D., Saner, F. (2019). Organ transplantation in the
modern era. BMC Anesthesiol, 19(32). https://doi.org/10.1186/
s12871-019-0704-z

Calne, R. (1994). The history and development of organ
transplantation: biology and rejection. Baillière's Clinical
Gastroenterology, 8(3), 389–397. https://doi.org/
10.1016/0950-3528(94)90026-4

Chang, E., Scudamore, H. C. & Chung, W. S. (2004). Transplantation: focus on kidney, liver and islet cells. Canadian Journal of Surgery: Journal Canadien de Chirurgie, 47(2), 122–129.

Dangoor, Y. J., Hakim, N. D., Singh, P. R. & Hakim, S. N. (2015). Transplantation: A Brief History. Experimental and Clinical Transplantation, 13(1), 1–5. https://doi.org./10.6002/ect.2014.0258

Jing, L., Yao, L., Zhao, M., Peng, LP. & Liu MY. (2018). Organ preservation: from the past to the future. Acta Pharmacologica Sinica, 39(5), 845–857. https://doi.org/10.1038/aps.2017.182

Rodrigue, J., Greene A. & Boggs, S. (1994). Current status of psychological research in organ transplantation. Journal of Clinical Psychology in Medical Settings., 1(1), 41–70. https://doi.org/10.1007/BF01991724

Watson, C. & Dark, J. (2012). Organ transplantation: historical perspective and current practice, BJA: British Journal of Anaesthesia, 108(1), 29–42. https://doi.org/10.1093/bja/aer384

**Chapter 4:**

ADInstruments. (n.d.). Isolated Organ. https://www.adinstruments.com/research/vitro/pharmacology-isolated-tissue-and-organs/isolated-organ

Alberta. (2020). Organ and Tissue Donation in Alberta. Government of Alberta. https://myhealth.alberta.ca/alberta/Pages/organ-and-tissue-donation-topic-overview.aspx

American Psychological Association. (2017). Ethical principles of psychologists and code of conduct. https://www.apa.org/ethics/code

Boettner, B. (2020). Next generation of organ-on-chip has arrived. https://news.harvard.edu/gazette/story/2020/01/human-body-on-chip-platform-may-speed-up-drug-development/

Cleveland Clinic. (n.d.). Organ Donation Facts & Info: Organ Transplants. https://my.clevelandclinic.org/health/articles/11750-organ-donation-and-transplantation.

Government of Canada. (2021). Research Ethics Board: About the Health Canada and Public Health Agency of Canada REB. https://www.canada.ca/en/health-canada/services/science-research/science-advice-decision-making/research-ethics-board.html

Knottenbelt, M. (2019). Three Benefits of Isolated Organ Research. ADInstruments. https://www.adinstruments.com/blog/three-benefits-isolated-organ-research.

LifeSource. (2021). Does My Race & Ethnicity Matter in Organ Donation? https://www.life-source.org/latest/does-my-race-ethnicity-matter-in-organ-donation/.

Liverman, C. T., Domnitz, S., & Childress. (2017). Opportunities for organ donor intervention research: Saving lives by improving the quality and quantity of organs for transplantation. National Academies Press. https://www.ncbi.nlm.nih.gov/books/NBK470918/.

Low, L. A., Mummery, C., Berridge, B. R., Austin, C. P., & Tagle, D. A. (2021). Organs-on-chips: into the next decade. Nat Rev Drug Discov, 20, 345–361. https://doi.org/10.1038/s41573-020-0079-3

McCall, V. (2021). The Secret Lives of Cadavers. Science. https://www.nationalgeographic.com/science/article/body-donation-cadavers-anatomy-medical-education.

National Kidney Foundation. (2016). Organ Donation and Transplantation Statistics. https://www.kidney.org/news/newsroom/factsheets/Organ-Donation-and-Transplantation-Stats.

Physicians Committee for Responsible Medicine. (n.d.). Donate Your Body to Science. https://www.pcrm.org/ethical-science/animal-testing-and-alternatives/donate-your-body-to-science

Shanti, A., Teo, J., & Stefanini C. (2018). In vitro immune organs-on-chip for drug development: A review. Pharmaceutics, 10(4), 278. https://doi.org/10.3390/pharmaceutics10040278

Statistics Canada. (2019). Data tables, 2016 census. https://www12.statcan.gc.ca/census-recensement/2016/dp-pd/dt-td/Rp-eng.cfm?TABID=2&Lang=E&APATH=3&DETAIL=0&DIM=0&FL=A&FREE=0&GC=0&GID=1341679&GK=0&GRP=1&PID=110563&PRID=10&PTYPE=109445&S=0&SHOWALL=0&SUB=0&Temporal=2017&THEME=120&VID=0&VNAMEE=&VNAMEF=&D1=0&D2=0&D3=0&D4=0&D5=0&D6=0

U.S. Government Information on Organ Donation and Transplantation. (2021). Organ Donation Statistics. https://www.organdonor.gov/statistics-stories/statistics.html.

Woods, B. (2017). It sounds futuristic, but it's not sci-fi: Human organs-on-chips. https://www.cnbc.com/2017/08/14/fda-tests-groundbreaking-human-organs-on-a-chip.html

Wyss Institute. (n.d.). Human organs-on-chips. https://wyss.harvard.edu/technology/human-organs-on-chips/


**Chapter 5:**

Bellini, M. I., & D'Andrea, V. (2019). Organ preservation: Which temperature for which organ? The Journal of International Medical Research, 47(6), 2323–2325. https://doi.org/10.1177/0300060519833889

Booster, M. H., Wijnen, R. M., van Hooff, J. P., Tiebosch, A. T., Peltenburg, H. G., van den Berg-Loonen, P. M., van Kroonenburgh, M. J., Verschuren, T., Hofstra, L., & Kootstra, G. (1993). The role of the spleen in pancreas transplantation. Transplantation, 56(5), 1098–1102. https://doi.org/10.1097/00007890-199311000-00010

Cochrane, A. D., Smith, J. A., & Esmore, D. S. (1991). The "domino-donor" operation in heart and lung transplantation. The Medical Journal of Australia, 155(9), 589–593. https://doi.org/10.5694/j.1326-5377.1991.tb93923.x

Corfield, J. (n.d.). Allograft. Encyclopedia Britannica. Retrieved May 15, 2021, from https://www.britannica.com/science/allograft

Cowled, P., & Fitridge, R. (2011). Pathophysiology of Reperfusion Injury. In R. Fitridge & M. Thompson (Eds.), Mechanisms of Vascular Disease: A Reference Book for Vascular Specialists. University of Adelaide Press. http://www.ncbi.nlm.nih.gov/books/NBK534267/

Goila, A. K., & Pawar, M. (2009). The diagnosis of brain death. Indian Journal of Critical Care Medicine : Peer-Reviewed, Official Publication of Indian Society of Critical Care Medicine, 13(1), 7–11. https://doi.org/10.4103/0972-5229.53108

Gorantla, V. S., Schneeberger, S., & Andrew Lee, W. P. (2010). Chapter 113—Principles of Hand Transplantation. In J. Weinzweig (Ed.), Plastic Surgery Secrets Plus (Second Edition) (pp. 729–736). Mosby. https://doi.org/10.1016/B978-0-323-03470-8.00113-7

He, B., Han, X., & Fink, M. A. (2018). Procurement of Abdominal Organs in Multi-Organ Donation in Deceased Donor. In Organ Donation and Transplantation—Current Status and Future Challenges. IntechOpen. https://doi.org/10.5772/intechopen.77308

HRSA. (2018, May 7). How Organ Donation Works. Organ Donor. https://www.organdonor.gov/about/process.html

Johns Hopkins. (n.d.). Face Transplant. Johns Hopkins Medicine. Retrieved May 16, 2021, from https://www.hopkinsmedicine.org/health/treatment-tests-and-therapies/face-transplant

Justiz Vaillant, A. A., Misra, S., & Fitzgerald, B. M. (2021). Acute Transplantation Rejection. In StatPearls. StatPearls Publishing. http://www.ncbi.nlm.nih.gov/books/NBK535410/

Kay, M. D., Hosgood, S. A., Harper, S. J. F., Bagul, A., Waller, H. L., & Nicholson, M. L. (2011). Normothermic Versus Hypothermic Ex Vivo Flush Using a Novel Phosphate—Free Preservation Solution (AQIX) in Porcine Kidneys. Journal of Surgical Research, 171(1), 275–282. https://doi.org/10.1016/j.jss.2010.01.018

Lanchin, M. (2012, November 27). Isabelle Dinoire: Life after the world's first face transplant. BBC News. https://www.bbc.com/news/magazine-20493572

Lanese, N. (n.d.). How Long Can Organs Stay Outside the Body Before Being Transplanted? Live Science. Retrieved May 15, 2021, from https://www.livescience.com/how-long-can-donated-organs-last-before-transplant.html

Manji, R. A., Menkis, A. H., Ekser, B., & Cooper, D. K. C. (2012). Porcine bioprosthetic heart valves: The next generation. American Heart Journal, 164(2), 177–185. https://doi.org/10.1016/j.ahj.2012.05.011

Medline Plus. (n.d.). Transplant rejection. MedlinePlus Medical Encyclopedia. Retrieved May 15, 2021, from https://medlineplus.gov/ency/article/000815.htm

Nasr, M., Sigdel, T., & Sarwal, M. (2016). Advances in

diagnostics for transplant rejection. Expert Review of Molecular Diagnostics, 16(10), 1121–1132. https://doi.org/10.1080/14737159.2016.1239530

Simko-Bednarski, E. (2021). World's first face and hands transplant gives New Jersey's Joe Dimeo a second chance at life. CNN. https://www.cnn.com/2021/02/03/us/face-and-double-hand-transplant/index.html

Tingle, S. J., Figueiredo, R. S., Moir, J. A., Goodfellow, M., Talbot, D., & Wilson, C. H. (2019). Machine perfusion preservation versus static cold storage for deceased donor kidney transplantation. Cochrane Database of Systematic Reviews, 3. https://doi.org/10.1002/14651858.CD011671.pub2

**Chapter 6:**

American Cancer Society | Information and Resources about for Cancer: Breast, Colon, Lung, Prostate, Skin. (2008, November 1). American Cancer Society. https://www.cancer.org/

Ang, G. C. (2005). History of skin transplantation. Clinics in Dermatology, 23(4), 320–324. https://doi.org/10.1016/j.clindermatol.2004.07.013

Barker, C. F., & Markmann, J. F. (2013). Historical Overview of Transplantation. Cold Spring Harbor Perspectives in Medicine, 3(4), a014977. https://doi.org/10.1101/cshperspect.a014977

Calne, R. (1994). The history and development of organ transplantation: biology and rejection. Baillière's Clinical Gastroenterology, 8(3), 389–397. https://doi.org/10.1016/0950-3528(94)90026-4

Chandak, P., & Callaghan, C. (2014). The immunology of organ transplantation. Surgery (Oxford), 32(7), 325–332. https://doi.org/10.1016/j.mpsur.2014.04.012

History of kidney transplantation. (2018, December 19). Edren.Org. https://edren.org/ren/unit/history/history-of-kidney-transplation/

Jain, A., & Bansal, R. (2015). Applications of regenerative medicine in organ transplantation. Journal of Pharmacy and Bioallied Sciences, 7(3), 188. https://doi.org/10.4103/0975-7406.160013

Stevens, S. (2016). Synthetic Biology in Cell and Organ Transplantation. Cold Spring Harbor Perspectives in Biology, 9(2), a029561. https://doi.org/10.1101/cshperspect.a029561

Timeline of Historical Events and Significant Milestones | Organ Donor. (2018, December 4). Organdonor.Gov. https://www.organdonor.gov/about/facts-terms/history.html

**Chapter 7:**
Azevedo, L. S., Pierrotti, L. C., Abdala, E., Costa, S. F., Strabelli, T. M., Campos, S. V., ... Marques, H. H. (2015).

Cytomegalovirus infection in transplant recipients. Clinics, 70(7), 515–523. https://doi.org/10.6061/clinics/2015(07)09

Babik, J. M., & Chin-Hong, P. (2015). Transplant Tourism: Understanding the Risks. Current Infectious Disease Reports, 17(4). https://doi.org/10.1007/s11908-015-0473-x

Balloy, V., Huerre, M., Latgé Jean-Paul, & Chignard, M. (2005). Differences in Patterns of Infection and Inflammation for Corticosteroid Treatment and Chemotherapy in Experimental Invasive Pulmonary Aspergillosis. Infection and Immunity, 73(1), 494–503. https://doi.org/10.1128/iai.73.1.494-503.2005

Biswas Roy, S., Panchanathan, R., Walia, R., Varsch, K. E., Kang, P., Huang, J., … Smith, M. A. (2018). Lung Retransplantation for Chronic Rejection: A Single-Center Experience. The Annals of Thoracic Surgery, 105(1), 221–227. https://doi.org/10.1016/j.athoracsur.2017.07.025

Black, C. K., Termanini, K. M., Aguirre, O., Hawksworth, J. S., & Sosin, M. (2018). Solid organ transplantation in the 21st century. Annals of Translational Medicine, 6(20), 409–409. https://doi.org/10.21037/atm.2018.09.68

Brennan, D. C. (2001). Cytomegalovirus in Renal Transplantation. Journal of the American Society of Nephrology, 12(4), 848–855. https://doi.org/10.1681/asn.v124848

Centers for Disease Control and Prevention. (2021, January 27). What is sepsis? Centers for Disease Control and Prevention. https://www.cdc.gov/sepsis/what-is-sepsis.html

Cukuranovic, J., Ugrenovic, S., Jovanovic, I., Visnjic, M., & Stefanovic, V. (2012). Viral Infection in Renal Transplant Recipients. The Scientific World Journal, 2012, 1–18. https://doi.org/10.1100/2012/820621

De Simone, B., Sartelli, M., Coccolini, F., Ball, C. G., Brambillasca, P., Chiarugi, M., … Catena, F. (2020). Intraoperative surgical site infection control and prevention: a position paper and future addendum to WSES intra-abdominal infections guidelines. World Journal of Emergency Surgery, 15(1). https://doi.org/10.1186/s13017-020-0288-4

Duncan, M. D. (2005). Transplant-related Immunosuppression: A Review of Immunosuppression and Pulmonary Infections. Proceedings of the American Thoracic Society, 2(5), 449–455. https://doi.org/10.1513/pats.200507-073js

Fabiani, S., Fortunato, S., & Bruschi, F. (2018). Solid Organ Transplant and Parasitic Diseases: A Review of the Clinical Cases in the Last Two Decades. Pathogens, 7(3), 65. https://doi.org/10.3390/pathogens7030065

Fernandez-Sabe, N., Cervera, C., Farinas, M. C., Bodro, M., Munoz, P., Gurgui, M., … Carratala, J. (2011). Risk Factors, Clinical Features, and Outcomes of Toxoplasmosis in Solid-Organ Transplant Recipients: A Matched Case-Control Study. Clinical Infectious Diseases, 54(3), 355–361. https://doi.org/10.1093/cid/cir806

Furtado, J. M., Smith, J. R., Belfort, R., Gattey, D., & Winthrop, K. L. (2011). Toxoplasmosis: A global threat. Journal of Global

Infectious Diseases, 3(3), 281. https://doi.org/10.4103/0974-777x.83536

Gavalda, J., Len, O., San Juan, R., Aguado, J. M., Fortun, J., Lumbreras, C., … Pahissa, A. (2005). Risk Factors for Invasive Aspergillosis in Solid-Organ Transplant Recipients: A Case-Control Study. Clinical Infectious Diseases, 41(1), 52–59. https://doi.org/10.1086/430602

Halawa, A., Abbas, F., El Kossi, M., Kim, J. J., Shaheen, I. S., Sharma, A., & Pararajasingam, R. (2019). Parasitic infestation in organ transplant recipients: a comprehensive review in the absence of robust evidence. Journal of The Egyptian Society of Nephrology and Transplantation, 19(2), 31. https://doi.org/10.4103/jesnt.jesnt_15_19

Ison, M. G., Hager, J., Blumberg, E., Burdick, J., Carney, K., Cutler, J., … Nalesnik, M. (2009). Donor-Derived Disease Transmission Events in the United States: Data Reviewed by the OPTN/UNOS Disease Transmission Advisory Committee. American Journal of Transplantation, 9(8), 1929–1935. https://doi.org/10.1111/j.1600-6143.2009.02700.x

Kalil, A. C., Sandkovsky, U., & Florescu, D. F. (2018). Severe infections in critically ill solid organ transplant recipients. Clinical Microbiology and Infection, 24(12), 1257–1263. https://doi.org/10.1016/j.cmi.2018.04.022

Khurana, S., & Batra, N. (2016). Toxoplasmosis in organ transplant recipients: Evaluation, implication, and prevention. Tropical Parasitology, 6(2), 123. https://doi.org/10.4103/2229-5070.190814

Kloc, M., & Ghobrial, R. M. (2014). Chronic allograft rejection: A significant hurdle to transplant success. Burns & Trauma, 2(1), 3. https://doi.org/10.4103/2321-3868.121646

Manuel, O., López-Medrano, F., Kaiser, L., Welte, T., Carrataià, J., Cordero, E., & Hirsch, H. H. (2014). Influenza and other respiratory virus infections in solid organ transplant recipients. Clinical Microbiology and Infection, 20, 102–108. https://doi.org/10.1111/1469-0691.12595

Mavrakanas, T. A., Fournier, M.-A., Clairoux, S., Amiel, J.-A., Tremblay, M.-E., Vinh, D. C., … Cantarovich, M. (2017). Neutropenia in kidney and liver transplant recipients: Risk factors and outcomes. Clinical Transplantation, 31(10). https://doi.org/10.1111/ctr.13058

Moreau, A., Varey, E., Anegon, I., & Cuturi, M.-C. (2013). Effector Mechanisms of Rejection. Cold Spring Harbor Perspectives in Medicine, 3(11). https://doi.org/10.1101/cshperspect.a015461

Nasr, M., Sigdel, T., & Sarwal, M. (2016). Advances in diagnostics for transplant rejection. Expert Review of Molecular Diagnostics, 16(10), 1121–1132. https://doi.org/10.1080/14737159.2016.1239530

Neofytos, D., Fishman, J. A., Horn, D., Anaissie, E., Chang, C.-H., Olyaei, A., … Marr, K. A. (2010). Epidemiology and outcome of invasive fungal infections in solid organ transplant recipients. Transplant Infectious Disease, 12(3), 220–229. https://doi.org/10.1111/j.1399-3062.2010.00492.x

Organ Donation Statistics. Organ Donor. (2021, April 2). https://www.organdonor.gov/statistics-stories/statistics.html.

Pappas, P. G., Alexander, B. D., Andes, D. R., Hadley, S., Kauffman, C. A., Freifeld, A., … Chiller, T. M. (2010). Invasive Fungal Infections among Organ Transplant Recipients: Results of the Transplant-Associated Infection Surveillance Network (TRANSNET). Clinical Infectious Diseases, 50(8), 1101–1111. https://doi.org/10.1086/651262

Patel, R., & Paya, C. V. (1997). Infections in Solid Organ Transplant Recipients. Clinical Microbiology Reviews, 10(1), 86-124.

Robert-Gangneux, F., & Darde, M.-L. (2012). Epidemiology of and Diagnostic Strategies for Toxoplasmosis. Clinical Microbiology Reviews, 25(2), 264–296. https://doi.org/10.1128/cmr.05013-11

Sagedal, S., Hartmann, A., Nordal, K. P., Osnes, K., Leivestad, T., Foss, A., … Rollag, H. (2004). Impact of early cytomegalovirus infection and disease on long-term recipient and kidney graft survival. Kidney International, 66(1), 329–337. https://doi.org/10.1111/j.1523-1755.2004.00735.x

Sandwijk, M. S. van, Bemelman, F. J., & Berge, I. J. M. T. (2013). Immunosuppressive drugs after solid organ transplantation. Netherlands Journal of Medicine, 71(6), 281–289.

Shoham, S., & Marr, K. A. (2012). Invasive fungal infections in solid organ transplant recipients. Future Microbiology, 7(5), 639–655. https://doi.org/10.2217/fmb.12.28

Schwartz, B. S., & Mawhorter, S. D. (2013). Parasitic Infections in Solid Organ Transplantation. American Journal of Transplantation, 13(s4), 280–303. https://doi.org/10.1111/ajt.12120

Silveira, F. P., & Husain, S. (2007). Fungal infections in solid organ transplantation. Medical Mycology, 45(4), 305–320. https://doi.org/10.1080/13693780701200372

Singh, N., & Limaye, A. P. (2015). Infections in Solid-Organ Transplant Recipients. Mandell, Douglas, and Bennett's Principles and Practice of Infectious Diseases, 3440–3452. https://doi.org/10.1016/b978-1-4557-4801-3.00313-1

Styczynski, J., Reusser, P., Einsele, H., de la Camara, R., Cordonnier, C., Ward, K. N., … Engelhard, D. (2008). Management of HSV, VZV and EBV infections in patients with hematological malignancies and after SCT: guidelines from the Second European Conference on Infections in Leukemia. Bone Marrow Transplantation, 43(10), 757–770. https://doi.org/10.1038/bmt.2008.386

Timsit, J.-F., Sonneville, R., Kalil, A. C., Bassetti, M., Ferrer, R., Jaber, S., … Van Delden, C. (2019). Diagnostic and therapeutic approach to infectious diseases in solid organ transplant recipients. Intensive Care Medicine, 45(5), 573–591. https:// doi.org/10.1007/s00134-019-05597-y

Unlu, O. (2015). Skin cancer in immunosuppressed transplant patients: Vigilance matters. World Journal of Hepatology, 7(4), 717. https://doi.org/10.4254/wjh.v7.i4.717

van Hal, S. J., Marriott, D. J. E., Chen, S. C. A., Nguyen, Q., Sorrell, T. C., Ellis, D. H., & Slavin, M. A. (2009). Candidemia following solid organ transplantation in the era of antifungal prophylaxis: the Australian experience. Transplant Infectious Disease, 11(2), 122–127. https://doi.org/10.1111/ j.1399-3062.2009.00371.x

Welte, T., Len, O., Muñoz, P., Romani, L., Lewis, R., & Perrella, A. (2019). Invasive mould infections in solid organ transplant patients: modifiers and indicators of disease and treatment response. Infection, 47(6), 919–927. https://doi.org/10.1007/ s15010-019-01360-z

Witter, A. R., Okunnu, B. M., & Berg, R. E. (2016). The Essential Role of Neutrophils during Infection with the Intracellular Bacterial PathogenListeria monocytogenes. The Journal of Immunology, 197(5), 1557–1565. https://doi.org/ 10.4049/jimmunol.1600599

## Chapter 8:

BC Transplant (2021). Deceased Donation. http:// www.transplant.bc.ca/health-info/organ-donation/deceased-donation

Beckman E. J. (2019). Management of the Pediatric Organ Donor. The journal of pediatric pharmacology and therapeutics : JPPT : the official journal of PPAG, 24(4), 276–289. https://doi.org/10.5863/1551-6776-24.4.276

By the Contributors to the C4 Article (Appendix 1) (2018). Current opinions in organ allocation. American journal of transplantation : official journal of the American Society of Transplantation and the American Society of Transplant Surgeons, 18(11), 2625–2634. https://doi.org/10.1111/ajt.15094

CIHI 2014: Deceased Organ Donor Potential in Canada. https://www.cihi.ca/sites/default/files/organdonorpotential_2014_en_0.pdf

COMMITTEE ON BIOETHICS (2013). Ethical controversies in organ donation after circulatory death. Pediatrics, 131(5), 1021–1026. https://doi.org/10.1542/peds.2013-0672

Donate-life (2021). Types of Donation. https://www.donatelife.net/types-of-donation/

Eshraghian, A. (2013). Religion, Tradition, Culture, and Solid

Organ Transplantation. Critical Care Medicine, 41(7), 134. doi: 10.1097/CCM.0b013e31828a2613

Institute of Medicine (2006). Organ Donation: Opportunities for Action. Washington, DC: the National Academies press. https://doi.org/10.17226/11642

Mayo Clinic (2021). Living-donor transplant https://
www.mayoclinic.org/tests-procedures/living-donor-
transplant/about/pac-20384787

Organ Donor Statistics (2021). https://www.organdonor.gov/
statistics-stories/statistics.html

Prison Legal News (2014). Prisoner Organ Transplants,
Donations Create Controversy Prisonlegalnews.org. https://
www.prisonlegalnews.org/news/2014/apr/15/prisoner-organ-
transplants-donations-create-controversy/.


Ro, C. (2021). Why The Global Kidney Exchange Remains
Controversial. Forbes. https://www.forbes.com/sites/
christinero/2019/12/15/why-the-global-kidney-exchange-
remains-controversial/.

Trindade, A. J., & Palmer, S. M. (2004). Current concepts and
controversies in lung transplantation. Respiratory care clinics of
North America, 10(4), 427–v. https://doi.org/ 10.1016/
j.rcc.2004.06.005

Van Meter C. H. (1999). The organ allocation controversy: how
did we arrive here?. The Ochsner journal, 1(1), 6–11.

WHO.-B (2021a). GKT1 Activity and Practices.
https:www.who.int/transplantation/gkt/statistics/en/

WHO. (2021b). Transplantation. https://www.who.int/
transplantation/organ/en/

## Chapter 9:

Aykas, A., Uslu, A., & Şimşek, C. (2015). Mass Media, Online Social Network, and Organ Donation: Old Mistakes and New Perspectives. Transplantation Proceedings, 47(4), 1070–1072. https://doi.org/10.1016/j.transproceed.2014.09.182

Boggi, U., Vistoli, F., Del Chiaro, M., Croce, C., Signori, S., Marchetti, P., Del Prato, S., Rizzo, G., & Mosca, F. (2004). Kidney and pancreas transplants in Jehovah's witnesses: ethical and practical implications. Transplantation proceedings, 36(3), 601–602. https://doi.org/10.1016/j.transproceed.2004.02.045

Chayko, M. (2016, April 16). What is Techno-social Life? The Superconnected Blog. https://superconnectedblog.com/2016/04/16/what-is-techno-social-life-2/

Gift of Life Donor Program. (n.d.). Sign up to save lives: Be an organ donor. https://www.donors1.org/learn-about-organ-donation/sign-up-to-save-lives/

Harel, I., Kogut, T., Pinchas, M., & Slovic, P. (2017). Effect of Media Presentations on Willingness to Commit to Organ Donation. Proceedings of the National Academy of Sciences, 114(20), 5159–5164. https://doi.org/10.1073/pnas.1703020114

Health Resource & Service Administration (HRSA). (n.d.). The organ transplant process. https://www.organdonor.gov/about/process/transplant-process.html

Health Resource & Service Administration (HRSA). (2021). Organ donation statistics. https://www.organdonor.gov/statistics-stories/statistics.html

Henderson, M. L., Adler, J. T., Van Pilsum Rasmussen, S. E., Thomas, A. G., Herron, P. D., Waldram, M. M., ... Segev, D. L. (2019). How Should Social Media Be Used in Transplantation? A Survey of the American Society of Transplant Surgeons. Transplantation, 103(3), 573–580. https://doi.org/10.1097/tp.0000000000002243

Jiang, X., Jiang, W., Cai, J., Su, Q., Zhou, Z., He, L., & Lai, K. (2019). Characterizing Media Content and Effects of Organ Donation on a Social Media Platform: Content Analysis. Journal of Medical Internet Research, 21(3). https://doi.org/10.2196/13058

Kindelan, K. (2019). a 19-year-old woman meets a 22-year-old stranger who donated his liver to her. GMA. https://www.goodmorningamerica.com/wellness/story/19-year-woman-meets-22-year-stranger-donated-62412411

Klug, L. A. (n.d.) Jewish funeral customs: Saying goodbye to a loved one. Jewish Federation of Greater MetroWest NJ. https://www.jfedgmw.org/jewish-funeral-customs-saying-goodbye-to-a-loved-one

Lindquist, K. A., MacCormack, J. K., & Shablack, H. (2015). The role of language in emotion: predictions from psychological constructionism. Front. Psychol. https://doi.org/10.3389/fpsyg.2015.00444

Major R. W. (2008). Paying kidney donors: time to follow Iran?. McGill journal of medicine : MJM : an international forum for the advancement of medical sciences by students, 11(1), 67–69.

McLuhan, M. (1964). Television: The Timed Giant. In Understanding Media: The Extensions of Man (pp. 364–364). essay, McGraw-Hill.

McLuhan, M., & Williams, R. (1978). Television: Technology and Cultural Form. Technology and Culture, 19(2), 259–261. https://doi.org/10.2307/3103751

Michalopoulos G. K. (2007). Liver regeneration. Journal of cellular physiology, 213(2), 286–300. https://doi.org/10.1002/jcp.21172

Morgan, S. E., Harrison, T. R., Long, S. D., Afifi, W. A., Stephenson, M. S., & Reichert, T. (2005). Family Discussions About Organ Donation: How the Media Influences Opinions About Donation Decisions. Clinical Transplantation, 19(5), 674–682. https://doi.org/10.1111/j.1399-0012.2005.00407.x

National Kidney Foundation. (2015), Living with one kidney. https://www.kidney.org/atoz/content/onekidney

National Kidney Foundation. (2017). Religion and organ donation. https://www.kidney.org/atoz/content/religion-organ-donation

National Kidney Foundation. (2019). What to expect after donation. https://www.kidney.org/transplantation/livingdonors/what-expect-after-donation

Paul Williams Independent Funeral Directors Ltd. (n.d.).
Jehovah's Witness funerals. https://
www.paulwilliamsfunerals.co.uk/funeral-services/religious-
funeral-services/jehovahs-witness-funerals

Rahman, R. (2011). Who, what why: What are the burial
customs in Islam? BBC News.

https://www.bbc.com/news/magazine-15444275

Ravelli, B., & Webber, M. (2019). Exploring sociology: A
Canadian perspective. Toronto:        Pearson.

YouTube. (2012, February 1). Noam Chomsky - The Purpose of
Education. YouTube. https://www.youtube.com/watch?
v=DdNAUJWJN08&t=374s.

 Zink, S., Zeehandelaar, R., & Wertlieb, S. (2005). Presumed vs
expressed consent in the US and internationally. Virtual Mentor,
7(9), 610-614. doi: 10.1001/virtualmentor.2005.7.9.pfor2-0509.

**Chapter 10:**

Altinörs, M. N. (2020). Future Prospects of Organ
Transplantation. In Organ Donation and Transplantation.
IntechOpen. https://doi.org/10.5772/intechopen.94367

CDC. (2019, January 30). Key Facts | Overview | Transplant
Safety | CDC. https://www.cdc.gov/transplantsafety/overview/
key-facts.html

Cooper, D. K. C., Dou, K.-F., Tao, K., Yang, Z., Tector, A. J., & Ekser, B. (2017, October 1). PIG LIVER XENOTRANSPLANTATION: A REVIEW OF PROGRESS TOWARDS THE CLINIC. https://www.ncbi.nlm.nih.gov/pmc/articles/PMC5030131/

Crapo, P. M., Gilbert, T. W., & Badylak, S. F. (2011). An overview of tissue and whole organ decellularization processes. Biomaterials, 32(12), 3233–3243. https://doi.org/10.1016/j.biomaterials.2011.01.057

Ekser, B., Li, P., & Cooper, D. K. C. (2017). XENOTRANSPLANTATION: PAST, PRESENT, AND FUTURE. Current Opinion in Organ Transplantation, 22(6), 513–521. https://doi.org/10.1097/MOT.0000000000000463

Health Resources & Services Administration. (2018b, May 7). Matching Donors and Recipients | Organ Donor. https://www.organdonor.gov/about/process/matching.html

Health Resources & Services Administration. (2021a, April). Organ Donation Statistics | Organ Donor. https://www.organdonor.gov/statistics-stories/statistics.html

Jing, L., Yao, L., Zhao, M., Peng, L., & Liu, M. (2018). Organ preservation: From the past to the future. Acta Pharmacologica Sinica, 39(5), 845–857. https://doi.org/10.1038/aps.2017.182

Peloso, A., Dhal, A., Zambon, J. P., Li, P., Orlando, G., Atala, A., & Soker, S. (2015). Current achievements and future

perspectives in whole-organ bioengineering. Stem Cell Research
& Therapy, 6(1), 107. https://doi.org/10.1186/s13287-015-0089-
y

Platt, J. L., & Cascalho, M. (2013). New and old technologies for
organ replacement. Current Opinion in Organ Transplantation,
18(2), 179–185. https://doi.org/10.1097/
MOT.0b013e32835f0887

Vanderpool, H. Y. (1999). Xenotransplantation: Progress and
promise. BMJ : British Medical Journal, 319(7220), 1311.

www.ingramcontent.com/pod-product-compliance
Lightning Source LLC
Chambersburg PA
CBHW032330210326
41518CB00041B/2047